V VETERINARY

M MEDICAL

S SCHOOL

A ADMISSION

R REQUIREMENTS

VETERINARY MEDICAL SCHOOL ADMISSION REQUIREMENTS

2010 Edition for 2011 Matriculation

Association of American
Veterinary Medical Colleges

PURDUE UNIVERSITY PRESS   WEST LAFAYETTE, INDIANA

Compiled by the Association of American Veterinary Medical Colleges;
Shaba Lightfoot, editor

Cover photograph courtesy of The University of Tennessee
Back cover photographs courtesy of:
1. University of Illinois at Urbana-Champaign
2. Cornell University
3. University of Wisconsin

Printed in the United States of America

ISBN 978-1-55753-555-9
ISSN 1089-6465

CONTENTS

FOREWORD

The profession of veterinary medicine offers a variety of exciting, enriching, and fulfilling career choices, including companion animal medicine, food animal medicine, public health, laboratory animal medicine, wildlife medicine, basic biomedical research and more. The Association of American Veterinary Medical Colleges (AAVMC) is pleased to provide this publication, Veterinary Medical School Admission Requirements (VMSAR), for students and their families considering applying to a College of Veterinary Medicine to help them understand exciting educational opportunities, and the application procedures and processes for our member Colleges of Veterinary Medicine. The Veterinary Colleges and Schools highlighted in this publication are accredited by the American Veterinary Medical Association. In addition, information is provided for our affiliate, non-AVMA accredited member s that are in the process of seeking accreditation.

VMSAR is published annually and provides the best concise, current and comparable information for those students interested in preparing for a career in veterinary medicine. There are many important factors to consider in preparing for an education in veterinary medicine including: special programs, financial aid, standardized tests, and the AAVMC Veterinary Medical College Application Service (VMCAS), as well as residency requirements for admission to the various colleges and schools.

VMSAR also provides current-year information on application requirements to all AAVMC member institutions. This information is presented in a way that makes it easy for prospective applicants to determine their best choices for the submission of applications. It is important for prospective applicants to determine where they have the best chance for admission based on state of residency. When that determination is made, the pre-veterinary medical course requirements are easier to manage and undertake with the greatest time efficiency.

Not all questions about applying to our colleges and schools will be available in this book. More information can be found on the college and school websites, which are provided in the heading for each institution. Additional information may be found on the AAVMC website; www.aavmc.org. Information may be obtained by personal contact with the appropriate office listed or by contacting the VMCAS Student and Advisor Hotline, either by email (vmcas@aavmc .org) or by its toll-free phone number (877-862-2740). Read all that is available in VMSAR and online first, and most questions will be answered.

AAVMC extends best wishes to all our readers with serious interests in the pursuit of a career in veterinary medicine. Careers in veterinary medicine are exciting, fulfilling, and rewarding in many ways. Veterinarians are held in high esteem by society and make significant contributions to improving the health and wellbeing of those they serve. We applaud and encourage your efforts to pursue a career in veterinary medicine, and wish you well in your pursuit of veterinary medical education.

Marguerite Pappaioanou
Executive Director, AAVMC

About the AAVMC

The Association of American Veterinary Medical Colleges (AAVMC) is a non-profit membership organization working to protect and improve the health and welfare of animals, people and the environment by advancing academic veterinary medicine. The Association was founded in 1966 by the deans of the then-existing 18 colleges of veterinary medicine in the United States and three in Canada. During the 1970s and 1980s, AAVMC's membership expanded to include departments of veterinary science in colleges of agriculture, and in the 1990s to include divisions or departments of comparative medicine.

Today, AAVMC provides leadership for the academic veterinary medical community, including in the United States all 28 colleges of veterinary medicine, nine departments of veterinary science, eight departments of comparative medicine, three other veterinary medical educational institutions, and internationally all five veterinary medical colleges in Canada, nine international colleges of veterinary medicine in Australia, Ireland, the Netherlands, New Zealand, and the United Kingdom, and four affiliate colleges of veterinary medicine.

Mission

AAVMC provides leadership for and promotes excellence in academic veterinary medicine to prepare the veterinary workforce with the scientific knowledge and skills required to meet societal needs through the protection of animal health, the relief of animal suffering, the conservation of animal resources, the promotion of public health, and the advancement of medical knowledge. AAVMC pursues its mission by providing leadership in:

- Advocating on behalf of academic veterinary medicine;
- Serving as a catalyst and convener on issues of importance to academic veterinary medicine;
- Providing information, knowledge and solutions to support members' work; and
- Building global partnerships and coalitions to advance our collective goals.

Strategic Goals

1. Lead efforts to review, evaluate, and improve veterinary medical education in order to prepare graduates with the competencies needed to address societal needs.
2. Lead efforts to increase the amount of veterinary research conducted and the number of graduates entering research careers.

3. Lead efforts to recruit a student body aligned with the demands for veterinary expertise.
4. Lead efforts to increase the number of racially and/or ethnically underrepresented in veterinary medicine (URVM) individuals throughout academic veterinary medicine.
5. Lead efforts to develop the next generation of leaders for academic veterinary medicine.
6. Strengthen AAVMC's capacity to better serve its members, partners, and other stakeholdersin advancing the AAVMC mission.

"URVMs are populations of individuals whose advancement in the veterinary medical profession have historically been disproportionately impacted by six specific aspects of diversity (gender, race, ethnicity, and geographic, socio-economic, and educational disadvantage) due to legal, cultural or social climate impediments." *Definition of Underrepresented in Veterinary Medicine (URVM)*, approved by the AAVMC Board of Directors, July 20, 2008.

ABBREVIATIONS

AAVMC	Association of American Veterinary Medical Colleges
AVMA	American Veterinary Medical Association
BA/BS	Bachelor of Arts or Bachelor of Science degrees
CLEP	College Level Examination Program
CVMA	Canadian Veterinary Medical Association
DVM/VMD	Doctor of Veterinary Medicine degree
GRE®	Graduate Record Examination
MCAT	Medical College Admission Test
MS	Master of Science degree
PhD	Doctor of Philosophy degree
SREB	Southern Regional Education Board
TOEFL	Test of English as a Foreign Language
VMCAS	Veterinary Medical College Application Service
VMD/DVM	Veterinary Medical Doctor degree
VMSAR	Veterinary Medical School Admission Requirements
WICHE	Western Interstate Commission for Higher Education

VETERINARY MEDICINE: OPPORTUNITIES AND CHOICES

Considered from the perspective of comparative medicine, veterinarians help animals and people live longer, healthier lives. They serve society by preventing and treating animal disease, improving the quality of the environment, ensuring the safety of food, controlling diseases transmitted from animals, and advancing medical knowledge. The Doctor of Veterinary Medicine degree can lead to diverse career opportunities and different lifestyles from a solo mixed-animal practice in a rural area to a teaching or research position at an urban university, medical center, or industrial laboratory. The majority of veterinarians in the United States are in private practice, although significant numbers are involved in preventive medicine, regulatory veterinary medicine, military veterinary medicine, laboratory animal medicine, research and development in industry, and teaching and research in a variety of basic science and clinical disciplines.

License to Practice

The DVM (or VMD) degree is awarded after 4 years of successful study at an accredited college of veterinary medicine. Graduate veterinarians are eligible to apply for a license to practice. Licensing is controlled by states and prov inces, each of which has rules and procedures for legal practice within its own jurisdiction. All require satisfactory completion of the national board exami nation, and most have other requirements, including additional tests and in terviews.

The spectrum of opportunities in Veterinary Medicine

Veterinarians may choose to become specialists in a clinical area or to work with particular species. The first step on the path toward specialization is usually an internship.

1) Clinical

Internship

Internships are 1-year programs in either small- or large-animal medicine and surgery. The most prestigious internship programs are at veterinary medical colleges or at very large private veterinary hospitals with board-certified veter inarians on staff. Since internships are usually at large referral centers, interns are exposed to a larger number of challenging cases than they would be likely to see in a smaller private practice.

Veterinary students in their senior year and veterinary graduates apply for internships through a matching program. Internship applicants and training hospitals rank each other in order of preference, and a computerized system matches each applicant with the highest-ranking teaching hospital that ranked the applicant. Academic performance in the veterinary professional curriculum, as well as recommendations from veterinary school faculty, is considered in the ranking of internship applicants.

Most veterinary interns in the United States receive a nominal salary, and their educational debts, if any, may be postponed in some governmentally subsidized loan programs. Veterinarians can often command a higher starting salary in private practice after completion of an internship. Also, an internship is the next step, after receiving the DVM degree, toward residency and board certification.

Residency Training

Veterinarians who complete internships or who have 2 years of private-practice experience are eligible to apply for residency programs. Residency training is more specialized than an internship. Currently, residency training is available in internal medicine, surgery, cardiology, dermatology, ophthalmology, exotic small animal medicine, pathology, neurology, radiology, anesthesiology, and oncology. The programs take 2 to 3 years to complete, depending on the nature of the specialty. Successful completion of a residency is required for certification by any of the veterinary medical specialty boards. Some residencies combine research and graduate study to lead to a master's degree.

Board Certification

Veterinary board certification and diplomate status are available for 20 specialties: anesthesiology, animal behavior, clinical pharmacology, dentistry, dermatology, emergency and critical care, internal medicine, laboratory animal medicine, microbiology, nutrition, ophthalmology, pathology, poultry medicine, private practice, preventive medicine, radiology, surgery, theriogenology (reproduction), toxicology, and zoological medicine.

2) Private and Public Practice

A significant percentage of veterinary graduates are engaged in private practice, either as an owner of a solo practice or, more likely, as a partner or associate in a group practice. Increasingly, veterinarians work together as a team, which allows a wider range of services to be provided.

Small-animal veterinarians focus their efforts primarily on dogs and cats but are seeing a growing number of pet birds and exotic animals such as reptiles.

Veterinarians specializing in large animals often place their emphasis on horses, cattle, or pigs, and work both on a farm-call and an in-clinic basis. A mixed-animal veterinarian works with all types of animals.

Some veterinarians obtain further specialization in such areas as diseases or disorders of the eyes of cats or reproduction difficulties in cattle.

Public practice provides a variety of opportunities at the national, state, county, or city levels. There are exciting career opportunities for veterinarians in food safety, public health, the military, animal disease control, research, and the care and maintenance of wildlife abound.

3) Industry

Veterinarians have many opportunities available to them in private industry, particularly in the fields of nutrition and pharmaceuticals. Assisting in the development of new products in the animal industry, conducting research for pharmaceutical companies, diagnosing disease and drug effects as pathologists, or safeguarding the health of laboratory animal colonies are all interesting career possibilities. Some veterinarians may be employed by zoos and aquariums and may act as consultants to wildlife preservation groups, game farms, or fisheries.

4) Conclusion

By the very nature of the comparative medical education that veterinarians receive, the many species of animals they care for and work for, and the wide variety of clientele served, the opportunities available to today's veterinarian are abundant.

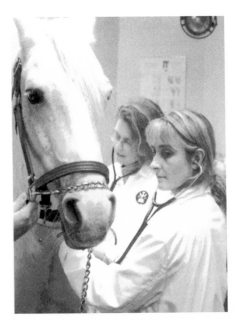

A Tufts University Cummings School of Veterinary Medicine student checks out a horse with advice from her professor. Photo courtesy of Andy Cunningham of the Tufts University Cummings School of Veterinary Medicine.

AAVMC MEMBER INSTITUTIONS AND THE ROLE OF ACCREDITATION

Veterinary Schools join the AAVMC as institutional or affiliate members. A key difference between these two membership categories is whether a college/school of veterinary medicine is accredited by the American Veterinary Medical Association's Council on Education (AVMA/COE). Only AVMA/COE accredited colleges of veterinary medicine may join AAVMC as an institutional (voting) member. Colleges of veterinary medicine that are not AVMA-accredited may join AAVMC as an affiliate member (non-voting) only. Several of AAVMC's affiliate members (Non-AVMA/COE accredited institutions) have entered into agreements with AAVMC institutional members for clinical training. It is important for prospective veterinary students to know the different implications of attending and/or graduating from AVMA/COE accredited vs. non-AVMA/COE accredited colleges of veterinary medicine as it pertains to educational options and eventually seeking and obtaining a license to practice veterinary medicine. AAVMC encourages its affiliate members to become AVMA/COE accredited.

Accreditation

The AVMA/COE accredits DVM or equivalent educational programs. Accreditation through the AVMA/COE assures that minimum standards in veterinary medical education are met by accredited colleges of veterinary medicine and that students enrolled in these colleges receive an education that will prepare them for entry-level positions in the profession. In the United States, graduation from an AVMA/COE accredited college of veterinary medicine is an important pre-requisite for application for licensure. Internationally, some veterinary schools have chosen to seek AVMA/COE accreditation in addition to accreditation by the competent authority in their own regions. AVMA/COE accreditation of international veterinary schools provides assurance that those programs of education meet the same standards as other similarly accredited schools.

Additionally, AVMA/COE accreditation assures:
- Prospective students that they will meet a competency threshold for entry into practice, including eligibility for professional credentialing and/or licensure;
- Employers that graduates have achieved specified learning goals and are prepared to begin professional practice;

- Faculty, deans, and administrators that their programs measure satisfactorily against national standards and their own stated missions and goals;
- The public that public health and safety concerns are being addressed; and
- The veterinary profession that the science and art of veterinary medicine are being advanced through contemporary curricula.

*Source: The source for this information and a site recommended for obtaining additional information is the following website: http://www.avma.org/education/cvea/about_accred.asp

Licensure

Licensure in the United States

In the United States, requirements for licensure are set by individual state regulatory boards. The North American Veterinary Licensing Exam (NAVLE) and any additional state exams must be taken by a graduate to become eligible for state licensure. The NAVLE, which is administered by the National Board of Veterinary Medical Examiners (NBVME), fulfills a core requirement for licensure to practice veterinary medicine in all jurisdictions in the United States and Canada. Mexico does not require NAVLE. In addition to the NAVLE, state regulatory boards will have other licensure requirements, which may include state-specific examinations.

To be eligible to take the NAVLE, applicants must have graduated from either an AVMA/COE- accredited college of veterinary medicine or a non-AVMA/COE accredited college (see following details).

Applicants who graduated from a non-AVME/COE accredited college must also have a certification of eligibility, which can come from one of two sources: the Educational Commission for Foreign Veterinary Graduates (ECFVG) Certification Program (http://www.avma.org/education/ecfvg/default.asp) or the Program for the Assessment of Veterinary Education Equivalence (PAVE) (http://www.aavsb.org/PAVE/PAVE Home.aspx).

All state regulatory boards accept the ECFVG certification, administered through the AVMA, as meeting in full or in part the educational prerequisite for licensure eligibility. At this time, 28 state regulatory boards also accept PAVE certification, which is administered through the American Association of Veterinary State Boards (AAVSB).

It is important to note that prerequisites for licensure eligibility and requirements for licensure vary amongst state regulatory boards and are subject to periodic modification.

Licensure Outside the United States

Mutual recognition arrangements apply to jurisdictions where there are AVMA/COE accredited schools. These specify that graduates of AVMA/COE accredited schools in the United States and Canada are permitted to obtain licensure to practice under terms no less favorable than graduates of schools accredited by the competent authority in that jurisdiction.

DECIDING WHERE TO APPLY

There are several factors, as well as the issue of accreditation, that an applicant must consider in identifying school(s) to submit an application for admissions. In addition to licensure issues, there may be economic, educational options, or other differences that students should consider in making decisions on where to apply. This book is intended to provide important information about AAVMC members to assist in informed decision-making for students considering applying to one or more veterinary colleges.

ALPHABETICAL LISTING OF AAVMC INSTITUTIONAL (AVMA/COE ACCREDITED) MEMBERS, BY COUNTRY

United States

Auburn University	Auburn, AL
Colorado State University	Fort Collins, CO
Cornell University	Ithaca, NY
Iowa State University	Ames, IA
Kansas State University	Manhattan, KS
Louisiana State University	Baton Rouge, LA
Michigan State University	East Lansing, MI
Mississippi State University	Mississippi State, MS
North Carolina State University	Raleigh, NC
Ohio State University	Columbus, OH
Oklahoma State University	Stillwater, OK
Oregon State University	Corvallis, OR
Purdue University	West Lafayette, IN
Texas A & M University	College Station, TX
Tufts University	North Grafton, MA
Tuskegee University	Tuskegee, AL
University of California, Davis	Davis, CA
University of Florida	Gainesville, FL
University of Georgia	Athens, GA
University of Illinois at Urbana-Champaign	Urbana, IL
University of Minnesota	St. Paul, MN
University of Missouri	Columbia, MO
University of Pennsylvania	Philadelphia, PA
University of Tennessee	Knoxville, TN
University of Wisconsin-Madison	Madison, WI
Virginia-Maryland Regional College of Veterinary Medicine	Blacksburg, VA
Washington State University	Pullman, WA
Western University of Health Sciences	Pomona, CA

Australia

Murdoch University	Murdoch, WA
University of Melbourne	Parkville, VIC
University of Sydney	Sydney, NSW

ALPHABETICAL LISTING OF AAVMC INSTITUTIONAL (AVMA/COE ACCREDITED) MEMBERS, BY COUNTRY

Canada

Université de Montréal	St. Hyacinthe, QC
University of Calgary	Calgary, AB
University of Guelph	Guelph, ON
University of Prince Edward Island	Charlottetown, PEI
University of Saskatchewan	Saskatoon, SK

Ireland

University College Dublin	Belfield, Dublin

The Netherlands

Utrecht University	Utrecht, Netherlands

New Zealand

Massey University	Palmerston North

United Kingdom

University of Edinburgh	Midlothian, Scotland
University of Glasgow	Glasgow, Scotland
Royal Veterinary College	London/Hertfordshire, England

ALPHABETICAL LISTING OF AAVMC AFFILIATE (NON-AVMA/COE ACCREDITED) MEMBERS, BY REGION

Caribbean

Ross University	St. Kitts, West Indies
St. George's University	Grenada, West Indies
St. Matthew's University	Grand Cayman Island, B.W.I.

Mexico

Universidad Nacional Autónoma de México	Mexico City, Mexico

Geographical Listing of Veterinary Schools and Directory of Admissions Offices

United States

Alabama

Office for Academic Affairs
College of Veterinary Medicine
217 Goodwin Student Center
Auburn University
Auburn AL 36849-5536

Office of Veterinary Admissions
College of Veterinary Medicine,
   Nursing and Allied Health
Tuskegee University
Tuskegee AL 36088

California

School of Veterinary Medicine
Office of the Dean-Student Programs
University of California
One Shields Avenue
Davis CA 95616

Western University of Health Sciences
Office of Admissions
College of Veterinary Medicine
309 East 2nd Street
Pomona CA 91766-1854

Colorado

Colorado State University
College of Veterinary Medicine and
   Biomedical Sciences
1601 Campus Delivery – Office of the
   Dean
Fort Collins CO 80523-1601

Florida

Admissions Office
College of Veterinary Medicine
P.O. Box 100125
University of Florida
Gainesville FL 32610-0125

Georgia

Admissions Department
Office for Academic Affairs
College of Veterinary Medicine
The University of Georgia
Athens GA 30602-7372

Illinois

University of Illinois
College of Veterinary Medicine
Office of Academic and Student Affairs
2001 South Lincoln Avenue,
   Room 2271g
Urbana IL 61802

Indiana

Admissions and Student Services Office
School of Veterinary Medicine
Lynn Hall, 1185
625 Harrison Street
Purdue University
West Lafayette IN 47907-2026

Iowa

Office of Admissions
College of Veterinary Medicine
2270 Veterinary Medicine
Iowa State University
P.O. Box 3020
Ames IA 50010-3020

9

Kansas

Office of Admissions
College of Veterinary Medicine
101 Trotter Hall
Kansas State University
Manhattan KS 66506-5601

Louisiana

Office of Veterinary Student and
   Academic Affairs
School of Veterinary Medicine
Louisiana State University
Skip Bertman Drive
Baton Rouge LA 70803

Massachusets

Office of Admissions
Cummings School of Veterinary
   Medicine
Tufts University
200 Westboro Road
North Grafton MA 01536

Michigan

Office of Admissions
College of Veterinary Medicine
F-104 Veterinary Medical Center
Michigan State University
East Lansing MI 48824-1314

Minnesota

Office of Academic and Student Affairs
College of Veterinary Medicine
108 Pomeroy Center
1964 Fitch Ave.
University of Minnesota
St. Paul MN 55108

Mississippi

Office of Student Admissions
College of Veterinary Medicine
P.O. Box 6100
Mississippi State University
Mississippi State MS 39762

Missouri

Office of Academic Affairs
College of Veterinary Medicine
W203 Veterinary Medicine Building
University of Missouri-Columbia
Columbia MO 65211

New York

Office of Student & Academic Services
College of Veterinary Medicine
S2-009 Schurman Hall
Cornell University
Ithaca NY 14853-6401

North Carolina

Student Services Office
College of Veterinary Medicine
North Carolina State University
4700 Hillsborough Street, Box 8401
Raleigh NC 27606

Ohio

Office of Student Affairs
College of Veterinary Medicine
Suite 127 Veterinary Medicine
   Academic Building
1900 Coffey Road
The Ohio State University
Columbus OH 43210-1089

Oklahoma

Office of Admissions
112 McElroy Hall
Center for Veterinary Health Sciences
College of Veterinary Medicine
Oklahoma State University
Stillwater OK 74078-2003

Oregon

Office of the Dean
Attention: Admissions
College of Veterinary Medicine
Oregon State University
200 Magruder Hall
Corvallis OR 97331-4801

Pennsylvania
Admissions Office
School of Veterinary Medicine
3800 Spruce Street
University of Pennsylvania
Philadelphia PA 19104-6044

Tennessee
Admissions Office
The University of Tennessee
College of Veterinary Medicine
2407 River Drive
Room A-104-C
Knoxville TN 37996-4550

Texas
Office of the Dean
College of Veterinary Medicine
and Biomedical Sciences
Texas A & M University
College Station TX 77843-4461

Virginia
Admissions Coordinator
Virginia-Maryland Regional College
of Veterinary Medicine
Blacksburg VA 24061

Washington
Office of Student Services
College of Veterinary Medicine
Washington State University
P.O. Box 647012
Pullman WA 99164-7012

Wisconsin
Office of Academic Affairs
School of Veterinary Medicine
2015 Linden Drive
University of Wisconsin-Madison
Madison WI 53706-1102

International

Australia
Murdoch International
Murdoch University
South Street
Murdoch 6150
Western Australia

University of Melbourne
Faculty of Veterinary Science
Corner Park Drive and
Flemington Road
Parkville
Melbourne 3010
Victoria Australia

Canada
Alberta
UCVM Admissions
TRW 2D03
3280 Hospital Drive NW
Calgary, AB T2N 4Z6

Montréal
Service des Admissions
Université de Montréal
C.P. 6205
Succursale Centre-Ville
Montréal Québec H3C 3T5 Canada

Ontario
Admissions Services
University Centre, Level 3
University of Guelph
Guelph Ontario N 1G 2W 1
Canada

Prince Edward Island
Registrar's Office
Atlantic Veterinary College
University of Prince Edward Island
550 University Avenue
Charlottetown PEI C1A 4P3
Canada

Saskatchewan

Admissions Office
Western College of Veterinary
 Medicine
University of Saskatchewan
52 Campus Drive
Saskatoon Saskatchewan S7N 5B4
Canada

Carribean

Ross University*
St. George's University*
St. Matthew's University*

England

Head of Admissions
Royal Veterinary College
Royal College Street
London NW1 0TU
England

Ireland

Veterinary Medicine Applications
UCD Admissions Office
Tierney Building
University College Dublin
Belfield, Dublin 4
Ireland

Mexico

Universidad Nacional Autónoma de
 México
Office of Undergraduate Studies
 (Division de Estudios Profesionales)
College of Veterinary Medicine
 (FMVZ)
Av. Universidad 3000
Circuito Interior
Delegacion Coyoacan
Mexico D.F. 04510

The Netherlands

Office for International Cooperation
Faculty of Veterinary Medicine
Utrecht University
Yalelaan 1
3584 CL Utrecht
The Netherlands

New Zealand

International Student Affairs
Massey University Veterinary School
Institute of Veterinary Animal and
 Biomedical Sciences
College of Sciences
Massey University
Private Bag 11-222
Palmerston North
New Zealand

Scotland

Admissions Office
Royal (Dick) School of Veterinary
 Studies
The University of Edinburgh
Easter Bush Veterinary Centre
Roslin EH25 9RG
Scotland

Director of Admissions & Student
 Services Manager
University of Glasgow Veterinary
 School
Bearsden Road
Bearsden
Glasgow G61 1QH
Scotland

LISTING OF SCHOOLS ACCEPTING NONRESIDENT/NONCONTRACT APPLICATIONS

United States	Number of Positions Available
Auburn University	Up to 15 positions; U.S. citizens only.
University of California	Limited number of positions.
Colorado State University	Up to 32 positions; international applicants considered.
Cornell University	Up to 43 positions; international applicants considered.
University of Florida	Not more than 15% of entering class; international applicants considered.
University of Georgia	Up to 10 positions.
University of Illinois	Up to 35 positions.
Iowa State University	Up to 50 positions, plus unfilled contract positions; international applicants considered.
Kansas State University	About 55% of class; international applicants considered.
Louisiana State University	Up to 22 positions.
Michigan State University	Up to 35 positions of entering class; international applicants considered.
University of Minnesota	Approximately 45% of entering class.
Mississippi State University	Up to 30 positions; international applicants considered
University of Missouri	Up to 40 to 50 positions.
North Carolina State University	18 positions.
Ohio State University	Up to 50 positions.
Oklahoma State University	Up to 22 positions.
Oregon State University	Up to 20 positions.
University of Pennsylvania	78 positions; international applicants considered.

Purdue University	30 positions; international applicants considered.
University of Tennessee	25 positions.
Texas A & M University	Up to 10 positions.
Tufts University	Minimum 40 positions; international applicants considered.
Tuskegee University	Up to 5 positions; international applicants considered.
Virginia-Maryland Regional College of Veterinary Medicine	Up to 15 positions.
Washington State University	Up to 25 positions; international applicants considered.
Western University of Health Sciences	Up to 100 positions for out-of-state applicants and up to 8 international positions.
University of Wisconsin International	Up to 20 positions.
University College Dublin	Up to 30 positions for international applicants.
University of Edinburgh	Up to 45 positions available for international applicants.
University of Glasgow	45 positions for international applicants.
Royal Veterinary College (London & Hertfordshire)	40 positions available for international applicants
University of Guelph	15 positions for international applicants.
Massey University	24 positions for international applicants.
University of Melbourne	50 positions for international applicants.
Murdoch University	Up to 32 positions for international applicants.
University of Sydney	Up to 35 positions for International applicants
University of Prince Edward Island	Up to 21 positions for international applicants.
Royal Veterinary College	Up to 30 positions for international applicants.

LISTING OF CONTRACTING STATES AND PROVINCES

Six Canadian provinces and 19 states in the United States have a veterinary school contract with one or more schools to provide access to veterinary medical education for their residents. The state or province, working through the contracting agency, usually agrees to pay a fee to help cover the cost of education for a certain number of places in each entering class. Residents from the contract states then compete with each other for those positions.

Some states contract with more than one school. For example, Arkansas contracts with 5 veterinary schools, and North Dakota has contracts with 6 schools. Connecticut, Rhode Island, Vermont, Nebraska, and the District of Columbia presently have no contracts, so all candidates from these places apply as nonresidents to veterinary schools of their choice.

The educational agreements between contracting agencies and veterinary schools differ. Under some contract arrangements, students pay in-state tuition; in others, they pay nonresident tuition. Some contract states require students to repay all or part of the subsidy that the state provided; others require veterinary graduates to return to practice in the state for a period of time. Applicants should be aware of their obligation to the state before agreeing to participate in a contract program.

Following is a list of states and provinces that have educational agreements with schools of veterinary medicine.

UNITED STATES

Arizona
Contracts through WICHE* with University of California, Colorado State University, Oregon State University, and Washington State University.

Arkansas
Contracts in past with Louisiana State University, University of Missouri, and Oklahoma State University. Contracts not all completed at time of printing; may be some changes.

Connecticut
Contracts with Iowa State University.

Delaware
Contracts with Oklahoma State University and the University of Georgia.

* WICHE = Western Interstate Commission for Higher Education (offices in Boulder, Colorado)

Hawaii
Contracts through WICHE* with University of California, Colorado State University, Oregon State University, and Washington State University.

Idaho
Contracts with Washington State University.

Kentucky
Contracts with Auburn University and Tuskegee University.

Maine
Contracts with Tufts University.

Montana
Contracts through WICHE* with University of California, Colorado State University, Oregon State University, and Washington State University.

Nebraska
Formal education alliance with Iowa State University.

Nevada
Contracts through WICHE* with University of California, Colorado State University, Oregon State University, and Washington State University.

New Hampshire
Contracts with Cornell University and Tufts University.

New Jersey
Contracts with Oklahoma State University, Tufts University, and Tuskegee University.

New Mexico
Contracts through WICHE* with University of California, Colorado State University, Oregon State University, and Washington State University.

North Dakota
Contracts with Iowa State University, Kansas State University, and the University of Minnesota. Contracts through WICHE* with the University of California, Colorado State University, Oregon State University, and Washington State University.

Puerto Rico
Cooperative agreement with University of Wisconsin.

South Carolina
Contracts with University of Georgia, Mississippi State University, and Tuskegee University.

South Dakota
Reciprocity with University of Minnesota. Contracts with Iowa State University.

Utah
Contracts through WICHE* with University of California, Colorado State University, Oregon State University, and Washington State University.

West Virginia
Contracts with University of Georgia, Tuskegee University, Mississippi State University, and Auburn University.

* WICHE = Western Interstate Commission for Higher Education (offices in Boulder, Colorado)

16

Wyoming
Contracts through WICHE* with the University of California, Colorado State University, Oregon State University, and Washington State University.

CANADA

Alberta
Contracts with University of Saskatchewan and University of Calgary.

British Columbia
Contracts with University of Saskatchewan.

Manitoba
Reciprocity with University of Minnesota. Contracts with University of Saskatchewan.

New Brunswick
Contracts with Atlantic Veterinary College at the University of Prince Edward Island and Université de Montréal.

Newfoundland
Contracts with Atlantic Veterinary College at the University of Prince Edward Island.

Nova Scotia
Contracts with Atlantic Veterinary College at the University of Prince Edward Island.

* WICHE = Western Interstate Commission for Higher Education (offices in Boulder, Colorado)

PROGRAMS FOR MULTICULTURAL OR DISADVANTAGED STUDENTS

The Association of American Veterinary Medical Colleges affirms the value of diversity within the veterinary medical profession. The membership is committed to incorporating that belief into their actions by advocating the recruitment and retention of underrepresented persons as students and faculty and ultimately fostering their success in the profession of veterinary medicine. The Association believes that through these actions society and the profession will be well served.

Many schools have programs designed to facilitate entry into, and retention by, veterinary programs nationwide. These programs are directed at several levels, from high-school students to the student who has already been accepted by a veterinary college. Most of these programs will accept students from every state, regardless of the school(s) to which an individual might eventually apply or attend.

Following is an alphabetical list of schools by state and a short explanation of their programs:

University of California

Program: Summer Enrichment Program

Description: a 6-week summer program. The purpose of this program is to increase the academic preparedness of disadvantaged students through science-based learning skills development, clinical education, individual advising, and student development.

Eligibility: Educationally and/or economically disadvantaged. Must have completed at least one year of college with a minimum science GPA of 2.50 and demonstrated interest in veterinary medicine.

Program dates: July–August.

Contact: Office of the Dean–Student Programs, School of Veterinary Medicine, University of California, One Shields Avenue, Davis CA 95616; telephone: (530) 752-1383.

Sponsorship: School of Veterinary Medicine, University of California-Davis.

Colorado State University

Program: Vet Prep

Description: a one-year academic program that serves as a bridge to the professional veterinary medical program for disadvantaged (cultural, social, economic) applicants who ranked high but were denied admission during the current admissions process. Limited to 7 students who upon successful completion are guaranteed admission to the veterinary program. Candidates are selected from the current regular admissions applicant pool.

Eligibility: disadvantaged students.

Contact: College of Veterinary Medicine and Biomedical Sciences, W102 Anatomy, Colorado State University, Fort Collins CO 80523; telephone: (970) 491-7051; email: DVMAdmissions@colostate.edu.

Sponsorship: College of Veterinary Medicine and Biomedical Sciences, Colorado State University.

Program: Vet Start

Description: an 8-year undergraduate and professional program for students who enter Colorado State from high school resulting in a bachelor's and a professional degree. Undergraduate and professional program scholarships are provided, and admission to the professional veterinary medical program is guaranteed upon successful completion of the undergraduate requirements. Mentoring, support services, and summer jobs are available to participants.

Eligibility: students who have a disadvantaged background (economic, cultural, or social) will be given special consideration. Students must be high-school graduates with fewer than 15 semester credits of college coursework. Selection is competitive. There are 5 positions per year for incoming freshman undergraduate students.

Program dates: begins fall semester; applications available online early December; application deadline first Monday in March.

Contact: College of Veterinary Medicine and Biomedical Sciences, Campus Delivery 1601, Colorado State University, Fort Collins CO 80523-1601; telephone: (970) 491-7051; email: ken.blehm@colostate.edu.

Sponsorship: College of Veterinary Medicine and Biomedical Sciences, Colorado State University.

Cornell University

Program: State University of New York Graduate Underrepresented Minority Fellowships

Description: all matriculating underrepresented minorities are eligible (not restricted by state residency).

Contact: Director of Student Financial Planning, College of Veterinary Medicine, S2-009 Schurman Hall, Cornell University, Ithaca NY 14853-6401; telephone: (607) 253-3766; www.vet.cornell.edu/public/financialaid/.

Program: Regents Professional Opportunities Scholarships

Description: a financial assistance program for New York residents who are underrepresented minorities. Must agree to work in New York for a time after graduation.

Contact: Director of Student Financial Planning, College of Veterinary Medicine, S2-009 Schurman Hall, Cornell University, Ithaca NY 14853-6401; telephone: (607) 253-3766; www.vet.cornell.edu/public/financialaid/.

Michigan State University

Program: Vetward Bound Program

Description: Vetward Bound offers different levels of programming, each with its own eligibility requirements. The program provides a review of basic science content, research and/or clinical experience, preparation for the GRE, veterinary experience, food and fiber animal experience, study strategy development, and field experiences. Level placement is determined by program staff and is based on educational background.

Eligibility: Economically and educationally disadvantaged first year undergraduate students through prematriculants into the professional degree program. Students selected to participate will meet HHS Health Careers Opportunity Program guidelines and Federal thresholds. An individual will be determined to be disadvantaged if he or she comes from a background that has inhibited the individual from obtaining the knowledge, skills, and abilities required to enroll in and graduate from a health professions school or comes from a family with an annual income below a level based on low income thresholds according to family size published by the Bureau of the Census, adjusted annually for changes in the Consumer Price Index, and adjusted by the Secretary for use in health professions programs.

Program dates: June–July.

Contact: Vetward Bound Coordinator, College of Veterinary Medicine, F113B Vet Med Center, Michigan State University, East Lansing MI 48824-1314; telephone: (517) 355-6521; email: vetbound@cvm.msu.edu.

Mississippi State University

Program: Board of Trustees of State Institutions of Higher Learning Veterinary Medicine Minority Loan/Scholarship Program

Description: a financial assistance program for Mississippi residents who are underrepresented minorities. The loan to service obligation is one year for each year of scholarship assistance, not to exceed four years.

Contact: Susan Eckels, Program Administrator, Mississippi Institutions of Higher Learning, 3825 Ridgewood Road, Jackson MS 39211-6453; telephone: (800) 327-2980.

North Carolina State University

Program: UNC Campus Scholarship Program—Graduate Student Component

Description: UNC General Administration funds this program. Eligibility is limited to new or continuing full-time doctoral students who have financial need and who are residents of North Carolina as of the beginning of the award period (as determined under the *Manual to Assist the Public Higher Education Institutions of N.C. in the Matter of Student Resident Classification for Tuition Purposes*). Individuals who have been accepted to a master's degree program in a department offering the doctoral degree and who intend, and will be eligible, to pursue doctoral studies at NC State after completion of the requirements for the master's degree are also eligible. The program provides up to $4,000 annually for North Carolina residents.

Contact: Director of Diversity Affairs, College of Veterinary Medicine, North Carolina State University, 4700 Hillsborough Street, Box 8401, Raleigh, NC 27606; telephone: (919) 513-6262; website: www.cvm.ncsu.edu.

Program: Diversity Graduate Assistant Grant

Description: Funded by the North Carolina State University Graduate School, recipients must be full-time, new or continuing students pursuing master's and doctoral degrees at North Carolina State University. The program provides up to $4,000 annually. Both resident and nonresident students are eligible to apply.

Contact: Director of Diversity Affairs, College of Veterinary Medicine, North Carolina State University, 4700 Hillsborough Street, Box 8401, Raleigh, NC 27606; telephone: (919) 513-6262; website: www.cvm.ncsu.edu.

Note: North Carolina residents are encouraged to apply for both programs. However, the annual maximum award for these grant programs is a combined $4,000. The grant is awarded on an annual basis. Awardees must reapply each year.

The Ohio State University

Program: Young Scholars Program

Description: this summer program is offered to seventh- through eleventh-grade students from Ohio. It provides hands-on science activities, academic enrichment exercises, and career exploration opportunities.

Eligibility: disadvantaged students recommended by their faculty.

Program dates: June to August each summer.

Sponsorship: the State of Ohio and The Ohio State University.

Program: Summer Research Opportunity Program

Description: this program is designed to promote the migration of minority undergraduate students into graduate research educational programs by providing them with summer research experiences. The student is provided with his or her individualized research problem by a faculty mentor and expected to carry that research through to publication.

Eligibility: the student must have completed 2 years of college work and have achieved at least a 2.50 cumulative GPA. The student must be an underrepresented minority or economically disadvantaged.

Contact: Graduate School, The Ohio State University, 230 North Oval Mall, Columbus OH 43210.

Sponsorship: the Big Ten Consortium for Institutional Studies.

University of Tennessee

Program: Veterinary Summer Experience for Tennessee High School Students

Description: The College of Veterinary Medicine offers an eight-week program that provides high school students an opportunity to gain experience working with veterinarians at a veterinary practice in their home towns for seven weeks during the summer. During the eighth week of this summer experience, students will be guests of the College of Veterinary Medicine on the campus of The University of Tennessee in Knoxville. Students will attend clinical rotations in the large animal, small animal and exotic animal (including zoo medicine) clinics in the Veterinary Teaching Hospital. Students will also attend special educational functions related to veterinary medicine.

Eligibility: To qualify for this summer program, a student must be a Tennessee resident and be enrolled as a senior, junior or sophomore in a Tennessee high school. Applicants must also have an interest in veterinary medicine as a potential career. Preference will be given to applicants who will contribute greatly to the diversity of the summer program and, potentially, to the verterinary profession. Students receive a financial stipend for satisfactory performance in the eight-week program.

Program dates: Summer

Contact: Dr. William Hill, The University of Tennessee, College of Veterinary Medicine, 2431 Joe Johnson Drive, 339 Ellington Plant Science, Knoxville TN 37996, telephone: (865) 974-5770. E-mail: vetsummer@utk.edu or wahill@utk.edu.

University of Minnesota

Program: Veterinary Leadership in Early Admissions for Diversity (VetLEAD)

Description: VetLEAD creates a pathway into the DVM program for high-ability students at under-represented serving partner schools, including Florida Agricultural and Mechanical University (FAMU).

Eligibility: Any high-achieving student enrolled the Animal Science program at FAMU may apply for an early admissions decision at the end of their second year of undergraduate studies. Eligible students have past experience working or volunteering in a veterinary related setting, a cumulative GPA of 3.4 with coursework consistent with required prerequisite courses, and strong letters of references.

Contact: Karen Nelson, Director of Admissions, dvminfo@umn.edu

Tuskegee University

Program: Summer Enrichment and Reinforcement Program (SERP) Description: this 6 -week preadmission program is designed to provide academic enrichment through effective learning strategies and mentorship to facilitate the entry of "at risk" students into the veterinary program and successful transition through the professional curriculum .

Description: this 8-week preadmission activity is designed to facilitate the entry of "at risk" students and provide the skills necessary for successful transition to the professional school.

Eligibility: participation is targeted to minority and disadvantaged students who have completed at least 3 years of college and all preveterinary prerequisites. Participation is restricted to persons who have applied to the DVM program in the College of Veterinary Medicine, Nursing, and Allied Health and who have been recommended by the Veterinary Admissions Committee for evaluation to the program.

Program dates: the summer before fall semester.

Contact: Associate Dean for Academic Affairs , College of Veterinary Medicine, Nursing and Allied Health, Tuskeegee University, Tuskeegee, AL 36088.

Sponsorship: this program is sponsored by a grant from the U.S. Department of Health and Human Services.

Program: Veterinary Science Training, Education and Preparation Institutes for Minority Students (Vet-Step I and II)

Description: Consists of 2 one-week programs designed to encourage high achieving minority students to consider veterinary medicine as a career choice. The program focus on progressive learning skills in reading comprehension, study skills, time-management, note-taking, medical vocabulary, etc.

Eligibility: Vet-Step I accepts 30 students from grades 9 and 10; Vet-Step II accepts students from Vet-Step I and from grade 12. Minority high school honor students interested in the biomedical sciences are strongly encouraged to apply.

Contact: Coordinator, Vet-Step Program, College of Veterinary Medicine, Nursing, and Allied Health, Tuskegee University, Tuskegee AL 36088, (334) 727-8309.

Sponsorship: U.S. Department of Health and Human Services.

Virginia-Maryland Regional College of Veterinary Medicine

Program: Multicultural Academic Opportunities Program

Description: a 10-week program providing opportunities to conduct scientific research; participate in clinical rotations within the veterinary teaching hospital; improve leadership, public speaking, and self-marketing skills; attend GRE preparatory classes; and learn about admission into graduate / professional school.

Contact: Admissions Office at Blacksburg campus.

Program: Summer Research Apprenticeship Program—College Park

Description: a summer research program providing research experience to veterinary and preveterinary students from diverse backgrounds, including economic hardship and underrepresented racial/ethnic groups. Projects may include assisting in the planning, preparation, and data collection for controlled experiments, clinical trials, or epidemiological investigations; researching disease processes; and performing literature searches.

Contact: Admissions Office at College Park campus.

Scholarship Opportunities: a limited number of scholarships are available to assist minority DVM students.

Washington State University

Program: Short-Term Research Training Program for Veterinary Students

Description: a 3-month summer program designed to promote interest in research by veterinary students. Emphasis is on a hands-on research project supervised by a faculty member with a research program. Stipends are provided.

Eligibility: WSU veterinary students or ethnic minority veterinary students from other U.S. colleges of veterinary medicine.

Program dates: 3 months in the summer dependent upon the summer vacation of the WSU College of Veterinary Medicine in which the veterinary student is enrolled.

Contact: Department of Veterinary Microbiology and Pathology, Washington State University, Pullman WA 99164-7040.

Sponsorship: The National Center for Research Resources.

University of Wisconsin

Program: Pre-College Enrollment Opportunity Program for Learning Excellence (PEOPLE)

Description: this program began in the summer of 1999 as a partnership between the Milwaukee Public Schools and the UW-Madison with a group of students who had just completed the ninth grade. New classes will be added each year, expanding to Madison area schools. The program is designed with a precollege track and a bridge program to undergraduate work and continues through a student's undergraduate career at University of Wisconsin-Madison. The main purposes are to promote academic preparation, increase enrollment in postsecondary institutions, and improve retention and graduation rates of minority and disadvantaged students.

Eligibility: students of one or more of the following ethnic heritages: African American, American Indian, Asian American, Hispanic/Latino. Other eligibility factors include economic disadvantage and current enrollment in or commitment to a college preparatory curriculum track.

Program dates: June–July summer residential programs and year-round nonresidential programs.

Contact: Assistant Vice Chancellor, 117 Bascom Hall, University of Wisconsin-Madison, Madison, WI 53706; or Associate Director, University of Wisconsin-Madison Undergraduate Admissions, Armory and Gymnasium, 716 Langdon Street, Madison, WI 53706.

Financial Aid Information

Financing your veterinary medical education requires careful planning, good money management skills, and a willingness to make short-term sacrifices to achieve long-range goals.

Many of you will apply for and receive some type of financial assistance during your undergraduate education. This will help you become somewhat familiar with the process, and to know that the rules and regulations governing programs can and do change periodically.

As a professional student, you will be entering a partnership with the financial aid office, which will require you to complete the appropriate financial aid forms accurately, meet required deadlines, and submit any additional information that may be requested. In return, the financial aid office will determine your aid eligibility and make awards based on the available programs. Your financial aid eligibility takes into account the cost of your education minus any other available resources. Amounts of assistance and the school policies for awarding assistance vary from one veterinary medical school to another and from year to year.

Any questions or concerns that you may have about this topic need to be directed to each of the appropriate financial aid offices to ensure that you receive accurate information and guidance.

Financing Your Veterinary Medical Education

Your education is one of the biggest investments you will make in your lifetime, and one of your most important goals should be to maximize the return on all of your investments. To reach this goal, you must take an active role in managing your financial resources. You need to understand and implement good financial practices. To get you started, here are some good financial habits you should adopt:

- Do not use credit cards to extend your lifestyle. Deciding not to use credit cards except in emergencies is one of the most important decisions you can make, and one that will reduce your stress while you are pursuing your education.
- Budget your money just as carefully as you budget your time. Contact a financial aid administrator to help you set up a budget that will be easy to follow.
- Distinguish between wants and needs. Before you make any purchase, you should ask yourself, "Do I need this, or do I want it?"
- Be a well-informed borrower. If you have not previously taken an active role in understanding the differences between various student loan programs, now is the time to do it. You need to know these differences in order to avoid high-interest loans and to borrow wisely.
- Borrow the minimum amount necessary in order to maximize the return on your educational investment.
- Be thrifty. Live as cheaply as you can. Remember, you are a student. You'll enjoy a more comfortable lifestyle once you are a DVM.
- Pay any interest that accrues on student loans if you can afford to do so, rather than let the interest accrue and capitalize. Any amount you pay while you're a student will save you money once you enter repayment.

What is the most important piece of advice for making the most of your educational investment? Don't live the lifestyle of a DVM until you have completed your education. Get in the habit of being thrifty. If you live like a DVM while you are in school, you may have to live like a student when you are a DVM.

FEDERAL LOAN PROGRAMS

	Subsidized Stafford Loan	Unsubsidized Stafford Loan
Lender	Financial or credit institution or eligible school	Financial or credit institution or eligible school
Financial Need	Yes	No
Citizenship Requirement	U.S. Citizen, U.S. National or U.S. Permanent Resident	U.S. Citizen, U.S. National or U.S. Permanent Resident
Borrowing Limits	$8,500/year; $65,500 aggregate undergraduate and graduate	Cost of attendance minus other aid; $189,125 aggregate undergraduate and graduate
Interest Rate	Fixed; capped at 6.8%	Fixed; capped at 6.8%
Interest Accrues School	No	Yes
Deferments	Yes	Yes
Grace Period	Yes	Yes

Perkins Loan	Health Professions Student Loan	Loan for Disadvantaged Students
Financial Aid Office	Financial Aid Office	Financial Aid Office
Yes	Yes	Yes
U.S. Citizen, U.S. National or U.S. Permanent Resident	U.S. Citizen, U.S. National or U.S. Permanent Resident	U.S. Citizen, U.S. National or U.S. Permanent Resident
$6,000/year; $40,000 aggregate undergraduate and graduate	Cost of attendance at participating school	Cost of attendance at participating school
5%	5%	5%
No	No	No
Yes	Yes	Yes
Yes	Yes	Yes

Information about Standardized Tests

Most veterinary medical colleges require one or more standardized tests: the Graduate Record Examination (GRE®) or the Medical College Admission Test (MCAT). For further information regarding test dates and registration procedures, contact the testing agencies listed below:

GRE Graduate Record Examination
P.O. Box 6000
Princeton NJ 08541-6000
(609) 771-7670 (Princeton, N.J.)
also: (510) 654-1200 (Oakland, Calif.)
www.gre.org
Individual school codes: see GRE booklet

MCAT Medical College Admission Test
MCAT Program Office
P.O. Box 4056
Iowa City IA 52243-4056
(319) 337-1357
www.aamc.org/students/mcat/

TOEFL Test of English as a Foreign Language
TOEFL/TSE Services
P.O. Box 6151
Princeton NJ 08541-6151
(609) 771-7100
www.toefl.org

VETERINARY MEDICAL COLLEGE APPLICATION SERVICE (VMCAS)

The Veterinary Medical College Application Service is a centralized application service sponsored by the Association of American Veterinary Medical Colleges. Applicants use VMCAS to apply to most of the AVMA accredited colleges in the United States and abroad.

VMCAS collects, processes, and ships application materials to veterinary colleges designated by the applicant, and responds to applicant inquiries about the application process. This service is the data collection, processing, and distribution component of the admission process for colleges participating in VMCAS. VMCAS, however, does not take part in the admissions selection process.

Twenty-five (25) of the twenty-eight (28) U.S. veterinary institutions participate in VMCAS, along with two (2) Canadian, two (2) Scottish, one (1) English, one (1) Irish, one (1) Australian, and one (1) New Zealand veterinary institutions. Application material deadlines, prerequisite courses, and other aspects of the admissions process differ from school to school. Applicants are responsible for being informed of all instructions provided by VMCAS and the associated member colleges. Questions about using VMCAS should be directed to the VMCAS Student & Advisor Hotline.

VMCAS
1101 Vermont Ave NW
Suite 301
Washington, DC 20005
Telephone (202) 682-0750
Toll-Free Student & Advisor Hotline (877) 862-2740
Fax (202) 682-1122
vmcas@aavmc.org
http://www.aavmc.org

VETERINARY MEDICAL SCHOOLS IN THE UNITED STATES

Auburn University

Office for Academic Affairs
Auburn University
College of Veterinary Medicine
217 Goodwin Student Center
Auburn AL 36849-5536
Telephone: (334) 844-2685
Email: admiss@vetmed.auburn.edu
www.vetmed.auburn.edu

The College of Veterinary Medicine at Auburn University is located in south central Alabama off Interstate 85 between Montgomery and Atlanta. The university is known for its friendly small-campus atmosphere despite having more than 24,000 students.

Veterinary medicine began as a department at Auburn in 1892 and became a college in 1907. Today it is situated on 280 acres one mile from the main Auburn campus. In addition, the college has a 700-acre research farm five miles from its campus. The college is fully accredited by the American Veterinary Medical Association.

Application Information

For specific application information (availability, deadlines, fees, and VMCAS participation), please refer to the contact information listed above.

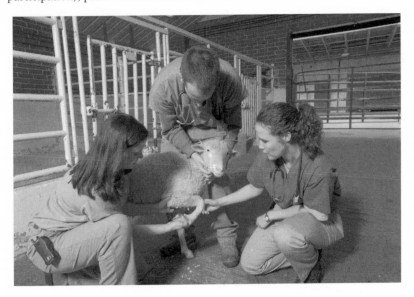

Residency implications: priority is given to Alabama residents. Auburn contracts with Kentucky for 40 positions and West Virginia for 2 positions. Up to 15 nonresident students are accepted.

Prerequisites for Admission

Course requirements and semester hours

	Written composition#	6
*	Literature#	3
	Fine Arts#	3
	Humanities/fine arts elective#	6
*	History#	3
	Social/behavioral science electives#	9
	Mathematics—precalculus with trigonometry#	3
	Biology I with lab	4
	Biology II with lab	4
	Fundamentals of chemistry with lab	8
**	Organic chemistry with lab	6
**	Physics	8
	Biochemistry	3
**	Science electives	6
##	Animal Nutrition	3

* Students must complete a 6-semester-hour sequence either in literature or in history.

** Organic chemistry, physics, and the two science electives must have been taken within 6 calendar years.

*** Science electives must be two of the following: genetics, microbiology, cell biology, comparative anatomy, histology, repro physiology, mammalian or animal physiology, parasitology, embryology, or immunology.

 # These requirements will be waived if the student has a bachelor's degree.

Will accept web based or correspondence course.

Required undergraduate GPA: a minimum grade point average of at least 2.50 on a 4.00 scale is required, with the minimum acceptable grade for required courses being C-minus. Applicants not classified as Alabama residents or contract students must have a minimum 3.00 GPA on a 4.00 scale. The mean grade point average of the most recent entering class was 3.53.

AP credit policy: must appear on official college transcripts and be equivalent to the appropriate college-level coursework.

Course completion deadline: prerequisite courses must be completed by June 15 prior to matriculation.

Standardized examinations: Graduate Record Examination (GRE®), general test, is required. The exam must have been taken within the previous 5 calendar years, and must be *received* no later than November 1 of the year of application.

Additional requirements and considerations
>   Animal/veterinary experience
>   Recommendations (3 required)
>   Academic advisor or faculty member
>   Employer
>   Veterinarian
>   Extracurricular and community service activities
>   Employment record
>   Narrative statement of purpose
>   Organic chemistry, physics and science electives must have been
>   completed within 6 calendar years

Summary of Admission Procedure

Timetable
>   VMCAS application deadline: Friday, October 1, 2010 12:00 PM
>   (noon) Eastern Time
>   Date interviews are held: February–March
>   Date acceptances mailed: March
>   School begins: August

Deposit (to hold place in class): none required.

Deferments: not considered.

Evaluation criteria
The 3-part admission procedure includes an objective evaluation of academic credentials, a subjective review of personal credentials, and a personal interview by invitation.

2008–2009 admissions summary

	Number of Applicants	*Number of New Entrants*
Resident	101	41
Contract*	103	38
Nonresident	555	15
Total:	759	94

Expenses for the 2009–2010 Academic Year

Tuition and fees
Resident	$13,402.00
Nonresident	
Contract*	$13,402.00
Other nonresident	$39,226.00

* For further information, see the listing of contracting states and provinces.

Entrance Requirements
Approximately half of the members of each class are Alabama residents. Auburn contracts with Kentucky for 40 positions and West Virginia for 2 positions. Kentucky students must verify their residency status with their Kentucky pre-vet advisor before October 1. They may contact the Kentucky Council on Postsecondary Education for additional information. West Virginia applicants should verify their residency by contacting Dr. Paul Lewis, Division of Animal & Nutritional Sciences at West Virginia University at (304) 293-3631, extension 4220 or by e-mail at grigs@wvu.edu before October 1.

Resident/contract applicants must be a documented resident of Alabama, Kentucky, or West Virginia and have a minimum grade point average of 2.50 on a 4.0 scale.

University of California

School of Veterinary Medicine
Office of the Dean—Student Programs
University of California
One Shields Avenue
Davis CA 95616
Telephone: (530) 752-1383
www.vetmed.ucdavis.edu

The University of California, Davis (UC Davis) campus is one of 10 campuses of the University of California. It is the largest campus, with 5,200 acres. The Davis campus is set between the Coast Range to the west and the towering Sierra Nevada to the east in the heart of the Central Valley. The campus is close to California's state capital and the San Francisco Bay Area but cherishes its small-town culture and security. Davis is surrounded by open space, including some of the most productive agricultural land in the state. The terrain is flat, and 50 miles of bike paths crisscross the city. Davis has earned the title "City of Bicycles." Winters in Davis are generally mild. Summers are hot and dry, usually in the low 90s, although some days it can exceed 100 degrees. Spring and fall weather is some of the most pleasant in the state. UC Davis is an outstanding research and training institution with over 30,000 undergraduate, graduate and professional students. The Davis campus has four undergraduate colleges, graduate studies in all schools and colleges, and professional programs carried out in the schools of Education, Law, Management, Medicine and Veterinary Medicine. The School of Veterinary Medicine is home of the William R. Pritchard Veterinary Medical Teaching Hospital, Veterinary Medicine Teaching and Research Center, California Animal Health and Food Safety Laboratory, UC Veterinary Medical Center-San Diego, Center for Companion Animal Health and Center for Equine Health. There are many other centers and innovative programs at UC Davis. The school is fully committed to recruiting students with diverse backgrounds.

Application Information

For specific application information (availability, deadlines, fees, and VMCAS participation), please refer to the contact information listed above.

Residency implications: priority is given to California residents. A small number of uniquely qualified nonresident applicants and WICHE applicants are accepted.

Prerequisites for Admission

Course requirements and quarter hours

General chemistry (with laboratory)	15
Organic chemistry (with laboratory)	6
Physics	6
General biology (with laboratory)	14
Systemic physiology*	5
Biochemistry* (bioenergetics and metabolism)	5
Genetics*	4
English composition and additional English	12
Humanities and social sciences	12
Statistics	4

* Upper-division courses equivalent to one semester or one quarter—labs not required.
Note: equivalent courses may vary in units and may also require other prerequisites. All lower division courses are full year courses on the semester system.

Required undergraduate GPA: a minimum grade point average of 2.50 on a 4.00 scale is required for both the required sciences (listed above) and cumulative college coursework. Applicants admitted in fall 2009 had a mean cumulative GPA of 3.53.

AP credit policy: credit and subject title must appear on official college transcripts.

Course completion deadline: all prerequisite courses must be completed prior to matriculation. Half of the required courses must be completed at the time of application.

Standardized examinations: Graduate Record Examination (GRE®), general test is required. The acceptable GRE test dates for applicants entering fall 2011 are October 1, 2005–October 1, 2010. The average GRE scores for the class admitted in 2009 are verbal 575, quantitative 712 and analytical writing 5.0.

Additional requirements and considerations
- Veterinary/animal experience
- Letters of evaluation (3)
- Personal statement of motivation/career goals
- Accuracy and neatness of application
- Interview

Summary of Admission Procedure

Timetable

> VMCAS application deadline: Friday, October 1, 2010 12:00 PM
> (noon) Eastern Time
> Date interviews are held: February to mid-March
> Date acceptances mailed: by April 1
> School begins: early September

Deposit (to hold place in class): none required.

Deferments: not considered.

Evaluation criteria	% weight
Grades	27
Test scores	23
Personal Statement/Essay/Animal and Veterinary Experience/References/Other	30
Interview	20

2009–2010 admissions summary

	Number of Applicants	Number of New Entrants
Resident	594	128
Contract*	88	1
Nonresident	453	4
Total:	1,135	133

Expenses for the 2009–2010 Academic Year

Tuition and fees

Resident	$27,045.00
Nonresident	$39,290.00
Contract student*	$39,290.00

* For further information, see the listing of contracting states and provinces. All nonresident and contract students are eligible for residency in California in one year.

Dual-Degree Programs

Combined DVM–graduate degree programs are available.
Visit our Veterinary Scientist Training Program information at
www.vetmed.ucdavis.edu/vstp.

Colorado State University

Colorado State University
College of Veterinary Medicine and Biomedical Sciences
1601 Campus Delivery – Office of the Dean
Fort Collins CO 80523-1601
Telephone: (970) 491-7052
Email: PreVetAdviser@colostate.edu (if you are an enrolled/future CSU student or you are a high school student)

DVMAdmissions@colostate.edu (if you are an undergraduate student, currently not attending CSU or you are a "prospective" applicant changing careers)
Web site: http://www.cvmbs.colostate.edu

Colorado State University is located in Fort Collins, a city of about 137,000 in the eastern foothills of the Rocky Mountains about 65 miles north of Denver. Fort Collins has a pleasant climate and offers many cultural and recreational activities. Many of the state's ski areas lie within a short driving distance, making some of the best skiing in the world accessible. The nearby river canyons and mountain parks are beautiful scenic attractions and provide opportunities for hiking, fishing, photography, camping, and biking.

The College of Veterinary Medicine and Biomedical Sciences is composed of 6 major buildings that house the departments of biomedical sciences, environmental and radiological health sciences, and microbiology, immunology, and pathology. The James L. Voss Veterinary Teaching Hospital, one of the world's largest and best-equipped, houses the clinical sciences department. This department boasts a variety of unique units, including the internationally acclaimed Robert H. and Mary G. Flint Animal Cancer Center, Animal Population Health Institute, Integrated Livestock Management Program, and Gail Holmes Equine Orthopaedic Research Center. The hospital attracts a large caseload and offers students a wide variety of clinical experiences.

Application Information

For specific application information (availability, deadlines, fees, VMCAS participation, and supplemental application requirements), please refer to the contact information listed above.

Residency implications: positions are allocated as follows: Colorado 75, WICHE contracts 29–48 (Arizona, Hawaii, Montana, Nevada, New Mexico, North Dakota, Utah, Wyoming), and nonsponsored 15-34. WICHE students must be certified by their states. Nonsponsored students can be from any state or country.

Prerequisites for Admission

Course requirements and semester hours

Laboratory associated with a biology course	1
Genetics	3
Laboratory associated with a chemistry course	1
Biochemistry	3
Physics (with laboratory)	4
Statistics/biostatistics	3
English composition	3
Social sciences and humanities	12
Electives	30

Required undergraduate GPA: No minimum requirement. The mean GPA for the 2009 matriculated class was 3.60 on a 4.00 scale.

AP credit policy: Must appear on official college transcripts.

Course completion deadline: transcripts with final grades, including all required courses, must be received by July 15 prior to matriculation.

Standardized examinations: Graduate Record Examination (GRE®), general test, is required and must be taken within the last five years prior to application. Scores must be received by October 1, 2010. Mean GRE scores for the 2009 matriculated class were verbal 522, quantitative 643, analytical 4.50.

Additional requirements and considerations
> Animal/veterinary/unique work experience
> Recommendations (3)—must be submitted electronically
>> Academic (academic advisor or college professor)
>> Employer
>> Veterinarian (at least 1 preferred)
> Essay
> Extracurricular and community service activities, leadership
> Quality of academic program (course load, challenging curriculum, honors)
> Contributions to diversity, unique attributes, extenuating circumstances

Summary of Admission Procedure

Timetable
> VMCAS Application deadline: Friday, October 1, 2010 10:00 a.m. Mountain Time
> School begins: late August

Deposit (to hold place in class): none required.

Deferments: not considered.

Evaluation criteria
> Grades, quality of academic program
> GRE® scores
> Animal/veterinary/other work experience
> Activities & achievements, community service
> Essay
> Letters of recommendation

2009–2010 admissions summary

	Number of Applicants	Number of New Entrants
Sponsored (Colorado)	266	75
Sponsored (WICHE)*	181	31
Nonsponsored	1,387	32
Total:	1,834	138

Estimated expenses for the 2010–2011 Academic Year

Tuition and fees (estimate, first 3 years)
Sponsored (Colorado & WICHE)	$18,858.00
Nonsponsored	$47,958.00

* For further information, see the listing of contracting states and provinces.

Dual-Degree Programs

Combined DVM–graduate degree programs are available (MBA/DVM, MPH/DVM, & DVM/PhD).

Special Programs

Food Animal Veterinary Career Incentive Program (FAVCIP)—program to admit up to 5 candidates per year who have strong backgrounds and interest in pursuing careers in food and production medicine.

For program eligibility, please see http://www.cvmbs.colostate.edu/cvmbs/FoodAnimalVetCareerIncentiveProgram.pdf.

Cornell University

Office of Student & Academic Services
College of Veterinary Medicine
S2-009 Schurman Hall
Cornell University
Ithaca, NY 14853-6401
Telephone: (607) 253-3700
Email: vet_admissions@cornell.edu
www.vet.cornell.edu/admissions

Cornell is located in Ithaca, a college town of about 30,000 in the Finger Lakes region of upstate New York, a beautiful area of rolling hills, deep valleys, scenic gorges, and clear lakes. The university's 740-acre campus is bounded on two sides by gorges and waterfalls. Open countryside, state parks, and year-round opportunities for outdoor recreation, including excellent sailing, swimming, skiing, hiking, and other activities, are only minutes away.

Ithaca is one hour by air and a four-hour drive from New York City, and other major metropolitan areas are easily accessible. Direct commercial flights connect Ithaca with New York, Boston, Chicago, Pittsburgh, Philadelphia, and other cities.

The tradition of academic excellence, the cultural vigor of a distinguished university, and the magnificent setting create a stimulating environment for graduate study. The curriculum differs from other programs in that it is interdisciplinary, small group learning early in the program and focuses on the student as the primary force in learning.

Application Information

For specific information about the application process visit our web site at http://www.vet.cornell.edu/education/DVM.htm. You may also subscribe to our free electronic newsletter at https://secure.vet.cornell.edu/admissions/application/inquiry.asp for application updates and current information about the College of Veterinary Medicine.

Residency implications: approximately 49 positions for New York State residents. Cornell contracts with New Hampshire.

Prerequisites for Admission

Course requirements and semester hours

English composition/literature*	6
Biology or zoology, full year with laboratory	6

* Three credits of literature may be satisfied by a course in public speaking.

Physics, full year with laboratory	6
Inorganic (general) chemistry, full year with laboratory	6
Organic chemistry, full year with laboratory	6
Biochemistry	4
General microbiology, with laboratory	3
Non-prerequisite elective credits needed	53

All prerequisites must have a letter grade of C– or better.

Required undergraduate GPA: No specific GPA requirement, but the grade range of those admitted tends to be 3.00–4.00.

AP credit policy: accepted for physics and inorganic chemistry with a score of 4 or higher.

Course completion deadline: all but 12 credits of the prerequisite coursework should be completed at the time of application, with at least one semester of any two-semester series underway. Any outstanding prerequisites must be completed by the end of the spring term prior to matriculation.

Standardized examinations: Graduate Record Examination (GRE®), general test, or the Medical College Admission Test (MCAT) is required. Official test scores must be received directly from ETS or AMA by Oct. 25. Test scores older than 5 years will not be accepted.

Additional requirements and considerations
    Animal/veterinary experience, knowledge, and motivation
    Recommendations/evaluations (3 required minimum)
        Academic advisor
        Animal-experience employers (1 required from each employer or experience)
        Nonveterinary work-related experiences (optional)
    Essay
    Extracurricular and/or community service activities

Summary of Admission Procedure

Timetable
    VMCAS application deadline: Friday, October 1, 2010 12:00 PM (noon) Eastern Time
    Supplemental application deadline: Oct. 25
    Information sessions at the college for admitted students and alternates: February/March
    Date acceptances mailed: January
    School begins: mid/late August

Deposit (to hold place in class): $500.00 (by April 15).

Deferments: considered on an individual basis, and ordinarily granted for illness or other situations beyond the control of the applicant.

Evaluation criteria
The admission procedure consists of 2 phases: an objective evaluation of academic credentials and a subjective review of the overall application.

	% weight
Grades	25
Test scores	25
Animal/veterinary experience	20
References, essay, quality of academic program, nonacademic activities, and noncognitive attributes	30

2009–2010 admissions summary

	Number of Applicants	Number of New Entrants
Resident	234	50
Contract*	10	0
Nonresident	657	42
Total:	901	92

Expenses for the 2009–2010 Academic Year

Tuition and fees

Resident	$26,500.00
Nonresident	
Contract student*	varies by contract
Other nonresident	$39,500.00

* For further information, see the listing of contracting states and provinces.

Dual-Degree Programs

Dual DVM–graduate degree programs are available. Our dual DVM/PhD degree students receive substantial financial incentives to complete both degrees. For more information visit http://www.vet.cornell.edu/OGE/dualDegree/

Leadership Program

The Leadership Program for Veterinary Students is a unique summer learning experience for veterinary students who seek to broadly influence the veterinary profession through a career in research. The program is an intensive, research-oriented learning experience that combines faculty-guided research with career counseling, student-directed learning, and a variety of professional enrichment activities.

Approximately twenty-five veterinary students from both the United States and abroad are accepted into the program each year.

Cornell also has a DVM/MPH with the University of Minnesota. More information can be found on the web site at: http://www.vet.cornell.edu/

University of Florida

Admissions Office
College of Veterinary Medicine
P.O. Box 100125
University of Florida
Gainesville FL 32610-0125
Telephone: 352-294-4272
Email: chaparro@ufl.edu
www.vetmed.ufl.edu

The University of Florida is located in Gainesville, a college town of approximately 100,000 in north central Florida, midway between the Gulf of Mexico and the Atlantic Ocean. Changes in season are marked, but winters are mild and permit year-round participation in outdoor activities.

The university accommodates about 40,000+ students with programs in almost all disciplines. The College of Veterinary Medicine is a component of the Institute of Food and Agricultural Sciences (which also includes Agriculture and Forest Resources and Conservation). It is also one of 6 colleges affiliated with the Health Science Center (the other 5 are Dentistry, Public Health and Health Professions, Medicine, Nursing, and Pharmacy).

The veterinary curriculum is a 9-semester program consisting of core curriculum and elective experiences. The core provides the body of knowledge and skills common to all veterinarians. The first 4 semesters concentrate primarily on basic medical sciences. Students are additionally introduced to physical diagnosis, radiology, and clinical problems during these years. The core also includes experience in each of the clinical areas. Elective areas of concentration permit students to investigate further the aspects of both basic and clinical sciences most relevant to their interests.

Application Information

For specific application information (availability, deadlines, fees, and VMCAS participation), please refer to the contact information listed above.

Residency implications: priority is given to Florida residents, and Florida has no contractual agreements. Nonresidents are considered in very limited numbers (not more than 15% of any entering class).

Prerequisites for Admission

Course requirements and semester hours

Biology (general, genetics, microbiology)	15
Chemistry (inorganic, organic, biochemistry)	19

Physics	8
Mathematics (calculus, statistics)	6
Animal Science (introduction to animal science, animal nutrition)	6
Humanities	9
Social sciences	6
English (2 courses in English composition)	6
Electives	at least 5

Required undergraduate GPA: a minimum GPA of 3.0 on a 4.00 scale. The class of 2012 had an overall mean science prerequisite GPA of 3.52.

AP credit policy: must appear on official college transcripts and be equivalent to the appropriate college-level coursework.

Course completion deadline: prerequisite courses must be completed by the end of the spring term prior to admission.

Standardized examinations: Graduate Record Examination (GRE®) is required. October 1, 2010 is the most recent acceptable test date for applicants to the class of 2014. Mean score for the class of 2013 was 1203.

Additional requirements and considerations
> Animal/veterinary experience
> Recommendations/evaluations (3 required)
>> Personal
>> Veterinarian
>> Academic advisor
> Honors and awards received
> Extracurricular activities
> Tracking Account (to download Additional Essay Form)

Summary of Admission Procedure

Timetable
> VMCAS application deadline: Friday, October 1, 2010 12:00 PM (noon) Eastern Time
> Date interviews are held: March
> Date acceptances mailed: April 1
> School begins: mid-August

Deposit (to hold place in class): none required.

Deferments: considered on an individual basis.

47

Evaluation criteria

The admission procedure consists of 3 parts: each applicant's file is reviewed; selected applicants are each interviewed for about 1 hour by 3 admissions committee members; final selection of new class takes place.

2009–2010 admissions summary

	Number of Applicants	Number of New Entrants
Resident	301	82
Contract	N/A	N/A
Nonresident	561	6
Total:	862	88

Expenses for the 2009–2010 Academic Year

Tuition and fees

Resident	$23,217.38
Nonresident	$44,192.58

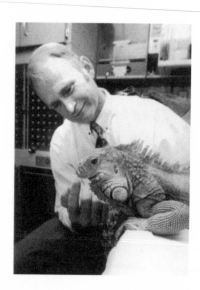

Not all of a veterinarian's patients are cuddly, especially for those specializing in wildlife and zoo medicine. Photo by Russ Lante, courtesy of University of Florida Health Science Center.

University of Georgia

Admissions Department
Office for Academic Affairs
College of Veterinary Medicine
The University of Georgia
Athens GA 30602-7372
Telephone: (706) 542-5728
www.vet.uga.edu/admissions
email: dvmadmit@uga.edu

The University of Georgia is located in Athens-Clarke County, with a population of over 100,000. Georgia's "Classic City" is a prospering community that reflects the charm of the Old South while growing in culture and industry (www. visitathensga.com). Athens is just over an hour away from the north Georgia mountains and the metropolitan area of Atlanta, and just over 5 hours away from the Atlantic coast.

In 1785, Georgia became the first state to grant a charter for a state-supported university. In 1801 the first students came to the newly formed frontier town of Athens. The University of Georgia has grown into an institution with 16 schools and colleges and more than 3,311 faculty members and 32,177 students.

Application Information

For specific application information (availability, deadlines, fees, and VMCAS participation), please refer to the contact information listed above.

Residency implications: Georgia retains up to 25 positions for contract students. Contracts are with Delaware (maximum 2), South Carolina (maximum 17), and West Virginia (maximum 6). The balance of those admitted are residents of Georgia or nonresident, noncontract applicants.

Prerequisites for Admission

Course requirements and semester hours

English (writing intensive)	6
Humanities and social studies	14
General biology with lab	8
Advanced biological science	8
Chemistry with lab	
Inorganic	8
Organic	8
Physics with lab	8
Biochemistry	3

Required undergraduate GPA: cumulative GPA of 3.00 or greater on a 4.00 scale or a combined score on the GRE® verbal and quantitative sections of 1200 or greater.

AP credit policy: must appear on official college transcripts and be equivalent to the appropriate college-level coursework.

Course completion deadline: prerequisite courses must be completed by the end of the spring term preceding entry.

Standardized examinations: Graduate Record Examination (GRE®), general test (including the analytical writing test), and the biology subject test must be completed within the 5 years immediately preceding the deadline for receipt of applications (October 1, 2010 12:00 PM (noon) Eastern Time). Test scores must be received by November 30 after the October 1 application deadline.

Additional requirements and considerations
>Animal experience
>Background for veterinary medicine
>Electronic Recommendations/evaluations (3 required)
>>Academic advisor/faculty member (required for graduate students)
>>Employer
>>Veterinarian
>Personal statement

Summary of Admission Procedure

Timetable
>VMCAS application deadline: Friday, October 1, 2010 12:00 PM (noon) Eastern Time
>Date acceptances mailed: mid-March
>School begins: mid-August. A required 5-day orientation will precede the start of classes.

Deposit (to hold place in class): $100.00; $500.00 for nonresident, noncontract students.

Deferments: one-year deferments considered for reasons such as completing a degree or for health problems.

Evaluation criteria
The admissions procedure includes a file evaluation. There are no interviews.
>Program of study
>Animal/veterinary experience
>References

Employment history
Personal statement
Extracurricular activities

2007–2008 admissions summary

	Number of Applicants	*Number Accepted*
Resident	187	76
Contract*	110	25
Nonresident	275	1
Total:	572	102

Expenses for the 2008–2009 Academic Year

Tuition and fees (approximate)
Resident	$14,230.00
Nonresident	
Contract*	$24,200.00
Nonresident	$38,430.00

Dual-Degree Programs

Combined DVM-graduate degree programs are available.
DVM-MPH Veterinarians in Public Health
DVM/PhD Veterinary Medical Scientist Training Program

University of Illinois

University of Illinois
College of Veterinary Medicine
Office of Academic and Student Affairs
2001 South Lincoln Ave., Room 2271G
Urbana IL 61802
Telephone: (217) 333-1192
Email: admissions@vetmed.illinois.edu

The University of Illinois is in Urbana-Champaign, a community of about 100,000 people located 140 miles south of Chicago. It is served by two airlines, 3 interstate highways, bus, and rail. The twin cities and university make a pleasant community with easy access to all areas and facilities. The university has about 42,000 students and more than 11,000 faculty and staff members. It is known for its high-quality academic programs and its exceptional resources and facilities. The university library has the largest collection of any public university and ranks third among all U.S. academic libraries. The university also has outstanding cultural and sports facilities and activities.

The College of Veterinary Medicine is located at the south edge of the campus. In addition to approximately 450 students, the college has about 100 graduate students plus a full complement of residents and interns. There are more than 100 full-time faculty with research interests in a variety of biomedical sciences and clinical areas. This research activity offers a broad variety of experiences for students. The college also offers students a dynamic, integrated core-elective curriculum to prepare for careers in almost any area of the profession.

Application Information

For specific application information (availability, deadlines, fees, and VMCAS participation), please refer to the contact information listed above.

Residency implications: priority is given to approximately 85 Illinois residents; approximately 35 nonresident positions are available.

Prerequisites for Admission

The academic requirements for application to the College of Veterinary Medicine can be met through one of two pathways: Plan A or Plan B. Those considering a career in veterinary medicine should have a good foundation in biological sciences and chemistry, including biochemistry, and should consider the specific courses listed in Plan A as the very minimum knowledge base for success in the curriculum.

* For further information, see the listing of contracting states and provinces.

Plan A

BS or BA degree in any major field of study from a regionally accredited college or university including the following courses (equivalent in content to those required for students majoring in biological sciences):

- a.   8 semester hours of biological sciences with laboratories
- b.   16 semester hours of chemical sciences, including organic, inorganic and biochemistry, with laboratories in inorganic and organic chemistry
- c.   8 semester hours of physics with laboratories

Plan B

Those applying without a bachelor's degree are required to present at least 60 semester hours from a regionally accredited college or university, including 44 hours of science courses. The minimum course requirements under Plan B are:

- a.   8 semester hours of biological sciences with laboratories
- b.   16 semester hours of chemical sciences, including organic, inorganic and biochemistry, with laboratories in inorganic and organic chemistry
- c.   8 semester hours of physics with laboratories
- d.   3 semester hours of English composition and an additional 3 hours of English composition and/or speech communication
- e.   12 semester hours of humanities and/or social sciences
- f. 12 semester hours of junior/senior-level science courses in addition to the requirements listed above

Applicants must have no more than 2 prerequisite courses to complete following the fall term in which they submit their application. All prerequisites must be complete by the end of the Spring 2011 term.

Required undergraduate GPA: a minimum cumulative GPA of 2.75 and a minimum science GPA of 2.75 on a 4.00 scale are required. The average statistics for students making it past Admissions Phase I in 2009 were 3.59 cumulative GPA, 3.49 science GPA, and 63% GRE® composite percentile.

AP credit policy: AP credit is allowed to meet the 8 s.h. physics prerequisite requirement if a student is awarded the full 8 s.h. AP credit is allowed for biology and chemistry if it is followed up by more advanced college-level courses in those science areas.

Standardized examinations: Graduate Record Examination (GRE®), general test, is required. Test must be taken by August 31 of the year of application, and scores may be no older than two years, i.e. Sept. 1, 2008-Aug. 31, 2010.

All 3 components of the exam must be completed as one exam. The higher composite score of the two most recent examinations will be used.

Additional requirements and considerations
    Animal and veterinary knowledge, motivation, and experience
    Recommendation/evaluation/suggestions
        Animal- and veterinary-experience employer
        Academic advisor/someone with knowledge of you as a learner
    Evidence of leadership, initiative, and responsibility
    Rigor of academic preparation

Summary of Admission Procedure

Timetable
    VMCAS application deadline: Friday, October 1, 2010 12:00 PM
        (noon) Eastern Time
    Informational program and required interviews: mid-February
    Date acceptances mailed: mid-late February
    School begins: late August

Deposit (to hold place in class): none required.

Deferments: considered on an individual basis by the Associate Dean for Academic and Student Affairs.

Evaluation criteria
A 3-part admission procedure is used. An academic evaluation and an application evaluation of veterinary, animal experience and personal qualities are followed by a personal interview.

Academic evaluation:
{
    GRE® test scores
    Science GPA
    Cumulative GPA
    Rigor of academic preparation

Nonacademic evaluation:
{
    veterinary-related experience, animal-related
        experience, community involvement,
        leadership, citizenship, and letters of
        recommendation

Interview

2008–2009 admissions summary

	Number of Applicants	Number of New Entrants
Resident	234	99
Nonresident	626	21
Total:	860	120

Expenses for the 2008–2009 Academic Year

Tuition and fees

Resident	$22,578.00
Nonresident	$41,042.00

Dual-Degree Programs

Combined DVM–M.S. and/or Ph.D. programs are available, and DVM/MPH with concurrent enrollment at University of Illinois at Chicago, School of Public Health.

Iowa State University

Office of Admissions
College of Veterinary Medicine
2270 Veterinary Medicine Iowa State University P.O. Box 3020
Ames IA 50010-3020 Telephone: (515) 294-5337
Toll free outside Iowa: (800) 262-3810
Email: cvmadmissions@iastate.edu
www.vetmed.iastate.edu

The Iowa State University College of Veterinary Medicine is located in the heart of one of the world's most intensive livestock-producing areas, which provides diverse food-animal clinical and diagnostic cases. A nearby metropolitan area and a regionally recognized referral veterinary hospital provide experience in companion-animal medicine and surgery. A strong basic science education during the first 2 years prepares veterinary students for a wide range of clinical experiences during the last 2 years. The College of Veterinary Medicine provides education in a wide variety of animal species and disciplines and allows fourth-year students to spend time with private practitioners, other colleges, research facilities, and in other educational experiences. Opportunities for research exist in the outstanding research programs in neurobiology, immunobiology, infectious diseases, and numerous other areas. The nearby National Animal Disease Center and the National Veterinary Services Laboratories provide additional research opportunities. The world's premier State Diagnostic Laboratory is part of the college and provides students with experience that is unmatched by any other veterinary college in the world. Graduates are highly sought after and can typically choose among 5 or 6 job offers. A career development and placement service is also provided.

Application Information

For specific application information (availability, deadlines, fees, and VMCAS participation), please refer to the contact information listed above.

Residency implications: priority is given to Iowa residents for approximately 60 positions. Iowa contracts on a year-to-year basis with North Dakota, South Dakota and Connecticut. Iowa also has a formal educational alliance with Nebraska. Remaining positions are available for residents of noncontract states or international students.

Prerequisites for Admission

Course requirements and semester hours

English composition[†]	6
General chemistry (1 year series w/lab)	7
Organic chemistry (1 year series w/lab)	7
Biochemistry	3
Physics (1 semester w/lab)	4
Biology (1 year series w/labs)	8
Genetics (Mendelian and molecular)	3
Mammalian anatomy and/or physiology	3
Oral communication	
(interpersonal, group or public speaking)	3
Arts, humanities, or social sciences	8
Electives	8

† English composition of one year or writing emphasis courses (may include business or technical writing).

Required undergraduate GPA: the minimum GPA required is 2.50 on a 4.00 scale. The most recent entering class had a mean GPA of 3.54.

AP credit policy: must be documented by original scores submitted to the university, and must meet the university's minimum requirement in the appropriate subject area. CLEP (College-Level Examination Program) credits accepted only for the arts, humanities, and social sciences.

Course completion deadline: It is preferred that prerequisite science courses be completed by the end of the fall term the year the applicant applies, and these must be completed with a C (2.0) or better to fulfill the requirement. However, up to 2 prerequisite science courses may be taken the spring term prior to matriculation. All other prerequisites must be completed by the end of the spring term prior to matriculation with a C (2.0) or better. Pending courses may not be completed the summer prior to matriculation. Pass–not pass grades are not acceptable.

Standardized examinations: Graduate Record Examination (GRE®), general test, is required.

Additional requirements and considerations
Recommendations (3 required). Academic advisors, veterinarians, and employers are suggested.

Summary of Admission Procedure

Timetable
>Application deadline: Iowa Residents: September 1, 2010
>All other applicants: Friday, October 1, 2010 12:00 PM (noon) Eastern
>>Time
>Date acceptances mailed: Approximately February 15
>School begins: late August

Deposit (to hold place in class): $500.00.

Deferments: considered on a case-by-case basis.

Evaluation criteria
The admission procedure consists of a review of each candidate's application
and qualifications:

1. Academic factors include grades, test scores, and degrees earned.
2. Nonacademic factors include essays, experience, recommendations,
   and personal development activities.
3. Interviews are conducted.

2008–2009 admissions summary

	Number of Applicants	Number of New Entrants
Resident	112	61
Contract*	108	38
Nonresident	557	49
Total:	777	148

Expenses for the 2010–2011 Academic Year

Tuition and fees
Resident	$16,624 (pending approval)
Nonresident	
Contract*	varies by contract
Other nonresident	$38,788.00 (pending approval)
Fees (approximate)	$895.00

* For further information, see the listing of contracting states and provinces.

Dual-Degree Programs

Combined DVM–graduate degree programs are available, including a DVM/
MPH and DVM/MBA.

Kansas State University

Office of Student Admissions
College of Veterinary Medicine
101 Trotter Hall
Kansas State University
Manhattan KS 66506-5601
Telephone: (785) 532-5660
Fax: (785) 532-5884
Email: admit@vet.k-state.edu
www.vet.k-state.edu

Kansas State University in Manhattan, Kansas, is located 125 miles west of Kansas City near Interstate 70. With a population of about 70,000 including KSU, Manhattan is in an area surrounded by many historical points of interest in a rich agricultural area of north central Kansas. Recreational activities abound in Manhattan and the surrounding area with fishing, boating, camping, and hunting among the favorites. Sporting events, theater, concerts, and excellent parks contribute to the many activities available. Kansans enjoy the 4 seasons, each of which brings its own special activities and events.

Kansas State University is on a beautiful 664-acre campus. The College of Veterinary Medicine opened in 1905. It is located on 80 acres just north of the main campus in 3 connected buildings.

Application Information

For specific application information (availability, deadlines, fees, and VMCAS participation), please refer to the contact information listed above.

Residency implications: to be eligible to be in the Kansas pool of applicants, the applicant must be a Kansas resident for tuition purposes at the time of application. Kansas accepts about 60 nonresident students per year. International applicants are considered. Kansas has a contract for students from North Dakota.

Prerequisites for Admission

Course Requirements and Semester Hours

Expository writing I and II	6
Public speaking	2
Chemistry I and II	8
General organic chemistry, with laboratory	5
General biochemistry	3
Physics I and II	8

Principles of biology or general zoology	4
Microbiology, with laboratory	4
Genetics	3
Social sciences and /or humanities	12
Electives	9

Science courses must have been taken within six years of the date of enrollment in the professional program.

Required undergraduate GPA: the required GPA to qualify for an interview is 2.80 on a 4.00 scale in both the prerequisite courses and the last 45 semester hours of undergraduate work. The most recent entering class had a mean prerequisite science GPA of 3.40.

AP credit policy: must appear on official college transcripts and be equivalent to the appropriate college-level coursework.

Course completion deadline: prerequisite courses must be completed by the end of the spring term of the year in which admission is sought.

Standardized examinations: Graduate Record Examination (GRE®), general test, scores are required by October 1, unless all prerequisites are completed at Kansas State University.

Additional requirements and considerations
> Animal/veterinary work experience and knowledge
> Employment record
> 3 evaluations required by nonfamily members, one a veterinarian, one academic or preprofessional advisor, one professor, or other professional.

Summary of Admission Procedure

Timetable
> VMCAS application deadline: Friday, October 1, 2010 12:00 PM (noon) Eastern Time
> Date interviews are held:
>> Kansas residents: mid-December
>> Nonresident: early January
>> New Mexico and North Dakota: February
> Date acceptances mailed: within 3 weeks after interview
> School begins: mid-August

Deposit (to hold place in class): $100.00 for Kansas residents, $250.00 for nonresident students.

Deferments: may be considered by Admissions Committee for extraordinary circumstances.

Evaluation criteria

A 4-part admission procedure is used, including evaluation of science grades, evaluation of all 3 GRE® scores, assessment of the application and narrative, and a personal interview.

Prerequisite science GPA	30%
Test scores	40%
Interview score including:	30%
References	
Animal/veterinary experience	

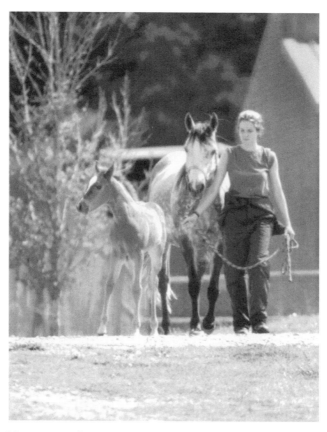

Veterinary students assist patients with rehabilitation schedules that include daily exercise. Photo courtesy of North Carolina State University College of Veterinary Medicine.

Leadership in college and community
Autobiographical essay

2009–2010 admissions summary

	Number of Applicants	Number of New Entrants
Resident	141	45
Nonresident	1,038	62
North Dakota	23	5
Total:	1,202	112

* For further information, see the listing of contracting states and provinces.

Expenses for the 2008–2009 Academic Year

Tuition and fees (subject to change)

Resident	$17,772.00
Nonresident	$40,104.00

* For further information, see the listing of contracting states and provinces.

Dual-Degree Programs

Combined DVM–graduate degree programs are available.
Combined DVM-MPH degree programs are available.

Early Admission Program

The Veterinary Scholars Early Admission Program is designed for those students having a genuine desire to enter the veterinary profession who attend Kansas State University with an ACT score of 29 or greater or an equivalent SAT score and who complete a successful interview during the fall semester of their freshman undergraduate year.

Louisiana State University

Office of Student and Academic Affairs
School of Veterinary Medicine
Louisiana State University
Skip Bertman Drive
Baton Rouge LA 70803
Telephone: (225) 578-9537
Fax: (225) 578-9546
Email: admissions@vetmed.lsu.edu
www.vetmed.lsu.edu

The Louisiana State University campus is located in Baton Rouge, which has a population of more than 500,000 and is a major industrial city, a thriving port, and the state's capital. Since it is located on the Mississippi River, Baton Rouge was a target for domination by Spanish, French, and English settlers. The city bears the influence of all three cultures and offers a range of choices in everything from food to architectural design. Geographically, Baton Rouge is the center of south Louisiana's main cultural and recreational attractions. Equally distant from New Orleans and the fabled Cajun bayou country, there is an abundance of cultural and outdoor recreational activities. South Louisiana has a balmy climate that encourages lush vegetation and comfortable temperatures year round.

The campus encompasses more than 2,000 acres in the southern part of Baton Rouge and is bordered on the west by the Mississippi River. The Veterinary Medicine Building, occupied in 1978, houses the academic departments, the veterinary library, and the Veterinary Teaching Hospital and Clinics. The school is fully accredited by the American Veterinary Medical Association.

Application Information

For specific application information (availability, deadlines, fees, and VMCAS participation), please refer to the LSU SM admissions website at www.vetmed.lsu.edu/admissions.

Residency implications: Louisiana contracts with Arkansas (9). Louisiana accepts up to 22 highly qualified nonresident applicants. Fifty-five seats are reserved for Louisiana residents.

Prerequisites for Admission

Course requirements and semester hours

General Biology	8
Microbiology (w/lab)[1]	4
Physics	6

General Chemistry	8
Organic Chemistry	3
Biochemistry[2]	3
English Composition	6
Speech Communication	3
Mathematics	5
Electives	20

[1]Lab component must accompany the microbiology lecture.
[2]Must have organic chemistry as prerequisite. For more details regarding prerequisites, visit the LSU SVM Admissions web site at www.vetmed.lsu.edu/admissions

Required undergraduate GPA: the minimum acceptable GPA for required coursework is 3.00 on a 4.00 scale. The mean GPA of the most recent entering class at the time of acceptance was 3.76.

AP credit policy: must appear on official college transcripts and be equivalent to the appropriate college-level coursework.

Course completion deadline: prerequisite courses must be completed by the end of the spring term preceding matriculation.

Standardized examinations: Graduate Record Examination (GRE®), general test, is required. The scores must be received no later than November 15. The average GRE combined verbal and quantitative score was 1143 for the class of 2013.

Additional requirements and considerations
    Animal/veterinary work experience
    Motivation, maturity, leadership skills
    Demonstrated communication skills
    Breadth of interests
    Entrepreneurial and business skills

Summary of Admission Procedure

Timetable
    VMCAS application deadline: Friday, October 1, 2010 12:00 PM
        (noon) Eastern Time
    Supplemental application deadline: November 16
    GRE® score submission deadline: November 16
    Date interviews are held: February/March*
    Date acceptances mailed: mid-March
    School begins: mid-August

*Interview invitations are extended to a select number of Louisiana, Arkansas, and out of state applicants as determined by the LSU SVM Admissions Committee.

Deposit (to hold place in class): $500.00 for nonresidents only.

Deferments: considered on a case-by-case basis.

Evaluation criteria
The approximate components of the evaluation scoring are:

    Objective evaluation:

GPA required courses	29%
GPA last 45 hours	18%
Test scores	18%

    Subjective evaluation:

Animal/veterinary experience, references (min. of 3 required, one by a veterinarian), essay, knowledge of profession, etc	15%
Personal interview	10%
Committee evaluation	10%

2009–2010 Admissions Summary

	Number of Applicants	Number of New Entrants
Resident	148	56
Contract*	27	9
Nonresident	467	22
Total:	642	87

Expenses for the 2009–2010 Academic Year

Tuition and fees (estimated)

Resident	$14,800.00
Nonresident	
Contract*	$14,800.00
Other nonresident	$39,000.00

* For further information, see the listing of contracting states and provinces.

Michigan State University

Office of Admissions
College of Veterinary Medicine
F104 Veterinary Medical Center
Michigan State University
East Lansing MI 48824-1314
Telephone: (517) 353-9793; fax: (517) 353-3041;
Helpline: (800) 496-4MSU (4678)
Email: admiss@cvm.msu.edu
www.cvm.msu.edu

Michigan State University's campus is bordered by the city of East Lansing, which offers sidewalk cafes, restaurants, shops, and convenient mass transit. The campus is traversed by the Red Cedar River and has many miles of bike paths and walkways. This park-like setting provides an ideal venue in which MSU's 46,500 students may enjoy outdoor concerts and plays, canoeing, and cross-country skiing. The older part of campus is situated north of the river. The ivy-covered buildings, some built before the Civil War and listed on the National Register of Historic Places, house five colleges, the student union, and 10 residence halls. South of the river are more recent additions to the campus, such as the Wharton Center for Performing Arts, the Jack Breslin Student Events Center, and several intramural sports facilities.

The college is a national leader in state-of-the-art technology and facilities. A lecture hall is equipped with a computer at each of the 116 work stations. These computers are part of a network that links all parts of the Veterinary Medical Center and allows instructors to receive immediate feedback on how well students understand the lecture material. The Veterinary Teaching Hospital has one of the largest caseloads in the country. Outstanding faculty are involved in teaching veterinary students, providing patient treatment and diagnostic services, and conducting veterinary research.

There are three new facilities that have been added in the past few years to our medical complex. They are the new Diagnostic Center for Population and Animal Health (DCPAH), the Center for Comparative Oncology, and the Matilda R. Wilson Pegasus Critical Care Center and the Training Center for Dairy Professionals. For information about these centers, please visit the links provided below.

http://www.dcpah.msu.edu/
http://cvm.msu.edu/news/insidecvm/archive/V30/V30N1.htm
http://cvm.msu.edu/vth/cco/index.htm
http://tcdp.cvm.msu.edu

Application Information

For specific application information (availability, deadlines, fees, and VMCAS participation), please refer to the contact information listed above.

Residency implications: priority is given to Michigan residents. Up to 35 positions are filled with nonresident and international applicants.

Prerequisites for Admission

Course requirements and semester hours
General education

English composition	3
Social and behavioral sciences	6
Humanities	6

Mathematics and biological and physical sciences

General inorganic chemistry (with laboratory)	3
Organic chemistry (with laboratory)	6
Biochemistry (upper-division)	3
General biology (with laboratory)	6
College algebra and trigonometry	3
College physics (with laboratory)	8
Nutrition	3
Genetics	3
Cell biology (eukaryotic)	3
Microbiology (with laboratory)	4

Required undergraduate GPA: 2.80 minimum cumulative GPA on a 4.0 scale; the mean cumulative GPA for the entering class (2009) was 3.66 on a 4.00 scale.

AP credit policy: AP credit(s) must appear on an official transcript and be equivalent to appropriate college-level coursework.

Course completion deadline: For those applying in 2010, prerequisite courses must be completed by August, 2011. Note: For those applying summer 2011 or later, all prerequisite courses must be completed by the end of spring semester in the year of matriculation.

Standardized examinations: The Graduate Record Examination (GRE®), general test, is required to be taken no later than September 30. For applicants to the class of 2015, the most recent acceptable GRE test scores are those of the September 30, 2010 exam. Test scores older than 5 years will not be accepted. For the class entering in 2009, average GRE scores were: 1176 combined verbal and quantitative. The Test of English as a Foreign Language (TOEFL) is required for applicants whose primary language is not English.

Additional Requirements and Considerations
- Evaluation of written application (including veterinary/research experience)
- Supplemental application
- Letters of recommendation (3 submitted by October 1 at noon EST time through VMCAS; 1 must be completed by a veterinarian)
- Interview (by the discretion of the Committee on Student Admissions

Summary of Admission Procedure

Timetable
- VMCAS application deadline: Friday, October 1, 2010 12:00 PM (noon) Eastern Time
- Electronic evaluations to VMCAS, Friday, October 1, 2010 12:00 PM (noon) Eastern Time
- GRE taken by September 30
- All transcripts submitted to MSUCVM by October 1 (postmarked date)
- International transcripts must be evaluated by a translation service such as World Education Services (WES), Josef Silny or the American Association of Collegiate Registrars and Admissions Officers, Foreign Education Credential Service (AACRAO). It is recommended that transcript(s) be submitted to the translation service at least one month prior to the deadline of October 1

Deposit (to hold place in class): (nonrefundable) $500.00 for residents; $1,000.00 for nonresidents.

Deferments: are rare.

2009–2010 admissions summary

	Number of Applicants	Number of New Entrants
Resident	231	74
Nonresident/International	692	32
Total:	923	106

Expenses for the 2008–2009 Academic Year

Tuition and fees

Resident	$21,678.00
Nonresident	$45,162.00

Early Admission Program

The Veterinary Scholars Admission Program has been established by the College of Veterinary Medicine in cooperation with the Honors College at Michigan State. This program provides an admission opportunity for students who wish to complete a bachelor's degree consisting of advanced, intellectually challenging, and scholarly studies in concert with their entry to the four-year professional veterinary medical degree program. Enrollment at MSU and membership in the Honors College are required to be eligible for this option. For information on Honors College membership, contact: Honors College, 103 Eustace Hall, Michigan State University, East Lansing, MI 48824; telephone (517) 355-2326; or visit their website at http ://www.msu.edu/unit/honcoll/.

Production Medicine Scholars Pathway

The Production Medicine Scholars Pathway to a Doctor of Veterinary Medicine degree will prepare students for a career in herd-based production medicine and agricultural veterinary practice. The pathway provides an early admission option for Michigan State University students planning to earn a baccalaureate degree in animal science with a concentration in production medicine. Successful applicants must have strong academic and non-academic credentials and a demonstrated interest in food animal production medicine and agricultural veterinary practice. Additional information about the pathway may be obtained from 1250 Anthony Hall, Department of Animal Science, Michigan State University, East Lansing, MI 48824 or visit the website www.canr.msu.edu/dept/ans/index.html.

Dual Degree Programs

Combined DVM – MPH degree program available
Combined online DVM/MS in Food Safety available

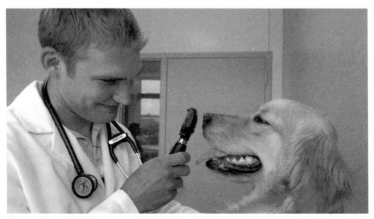

Photograph by Nat Lam.

University of Minnesota

Office of Academic and Student Affairs
College of Veterinary Medicine
108 Pomeroy Center
1964 Fitch Ave.
University of Minnesota
St. Paul MN 55108
Telephone: (612) 624-4747
Email: dvminfo@umn.edu
www.cvm.umn.edu

The University of Minnesota's College of Veterinary Medicine is located on the 540-acre St. Paul campus. Students enjoy a small-campus atmosphere as well as the academic, cultural, social, and recreational opportunities of a major university and large metropolitan area. Cultural life includes world-renowned institutions and a rich local mix of theater, music, and arts organizations. The Twin Cities is home to the state capital and the headquarters of many diverse major corporations. Minneapolis and St. Paul consistently rank near the top on quality-of-life and residential satisfaction ratings.

The College of Veterinary Medicine blends cornfields with biotechnology and cow barns with state-of-the-art diagnostic laboratories. The college provides contemporary facilities, including the Veterinary Medical Center, a new equine center, and the Raptor Center, which in 1988 became the world's first facility designed specifically for birds of prey. The educational opportunities extend beyond the campus to include farms throughout Minnesota and around the world. Students are given opportunities to learn about the practice of contemporary veterinary medicine through externships, clinical rotations, and first-hand experiences with practitioners.

Application Information

For specific application information (availability, deadlines, fees, and VMCAS participation), please refer to the contact information listed above.

Residency implications: first priority is given to residents of Minnesota and residents of states/provinces with which a reciprocity or contract agreement exists (North Dakota, South Dakota, Manitoba). Residents of other states are encouraged to apply. International applicants are only considered if their preveterinary courses have been completed at a U.S. college or university.

Prerequisites for Admission

Course requirements and semester hours

Freshman English, communication	6–9
Mathematics	3–5
Chemistry (with laboratory)	
General inorganic	8–12
General organic*	5–10
Biology (with laboratory)	3–5
Zoology/animal biology (with laboratory)	3–5
Physics (with laboratory)	8–12
Biochemistry	3–5
Genetics	3–5
Microbiology (with laboratory)	3–5
Liberal education	12–18

* Two quarters with one laboratory or one semester with laboratory

A minimum of 4 courses from the following areas of study: anthropology, art, economics, geography, history, humanities, literature (including foreign language literature), music, political science, psychology, public speaking or small group (interpersonal) communication, social science, sociology, theater.

Required undergraduate GPA: 2.75 minimum GPA required. The class of 2013 had a mean GPA of 3.55 (on a 4.00 scale) for required courses and 3.67 for the last 60 quarter-hour or 45 semester-hour credits of coursework prior to admission.

AP credit policy: must appear on official college transcripts and be equivalent to the appropriate college-level coursework.

Course completion deadline: prerequisite courses must be completed by the end of the spring term (not later than June 15) of the academic year in which application is made.

Standardized examinations: Graduate Record Examination (GRE®), general test, is required and must be taken by September 1 with results received by September 30. The mean combined score for the verbal and quantitative sections of the GRE for the class entering in fall 2009 was 1150.

Summary of Admission Procedure

Timetable

VMCAS application deadline: Friday, October 1, 2010 12:00 PM (noon) Eastern Time
Date acceptances mailed: mid-March
School begins: early September

Deposit (to hold place in class): $250.00.

Deferments: can be requested for special circumstances that warrant a 1-year delay in admission.

Evaluation criteria
    Objective measures of educational background
        GPA in required courses
        GPA in recent courses
        Test scores
    Behavioral interviews
    Subjective measures of personal experience
        Employment record
        Extracurricular and/or community service activities
        Leadership abilities
        References
        Maturity/reliability
        Animal/veterinary knowledge, experience, and interest

2008–2009 admissions summary

	Number of Applicants	Number of New Entrants
Resident*	219	61
Nonresident	864	36
Total:	1,153	97

The figures for new entrants include students taking delayed admission from the previous year.

*Includes residents of North and South Dakota and Manitoba.

Expenses for the 2009–2010 Academic Year

Tuition and fees
    Residents $22,146.00
    Nonresidents $42,190.00
* Additional fees apply

Mississippi State University

Office of Student Admissions
College of Veterinary Medicine
P.O. Box 6100
Mississippi State University
Mississippi State MS 39762
Telephone: (662) 325-9065
Email: MSU-CVMAdmissions@cvm.msstate.edu
www.cvm.msstate.edu

Starkville is home to more than 18,500 MSU students and their Bulldogs. Starkville is located in northeast central Mississippi and has a population of 22,000. Being a land-grant university, MSU is green and beautifully landscaped. The university includes 9 farms scattered throughout the state. The College of Veterinary Medicine (the Wise Center) was completed in 1982. The college includes 620 rooms on 8 acres, or 360,000 square feet, under one roof.

The curriculum of the MSU-CVM is divided into 2 phases: Phase 1 (freshman and sophomore years) and Phase 2 (junior and senior years).

- Year 1 uses foundation courses to expose the student to important medical concepts and address multidisciplinary problems.

- Year 2 is devoted to the study of clinical diseases and abnormalities of various animal species. Surgery labs begin in the second year.

- Year 3 is comprised of clinical rotations in the College's Animal Health Center, Referral/Emergency Clinic in Jackson, MS, the large animal ambulatory service, and elective courses.

- Year 4 is largely experiential and offers the student the opportunity, once required courses have been scheduled, to select among approved experiences in advanced clinical rotations, elective courses, or externships.

The first 3 years of the curriculum are 9–10 months in length, while the fourth year is 12 months.

Application Information

For specific application information (availability, deadlines, fees, and VMCAS participation), please refer to the contact information listed above.

Residency implications: Mississippi accepts 35–40 nonresident students and has 5 contract positions with South Carolina and West Virginia.

Prerequisites for Admission

Course requirements and semester hours

English composition	6
Speech or Technical Writing	3
Mathematics (college algebra or higher) *	6
General biology with laboraties	8
Microbiology with laboratory*	4
General chemistry with laboratories*	8
Organic chemistry with laboratories*	8
Biochemistry*	3
Physics (may be trig-based) *	6
Advanced (upper level) science electives*	12
Humanities, fine arts, social and behavioral sciences	15

* Science and mathematics courses must be completed or updated within six calendar years prior to the anticipated date of enrollment.

Required undergraduate GPA: a minimum GPA of 2.8 on a 4.0 scale overall and in required math/science courses. Minimum GPA must be maintained throughout the application process. The class of 2013 has an average undergraduate GPA of 3.56.

No grade lower than a C- is acceptable in any required course.

No course taken more than two times in pursuit of an acceptable grade may be used to meet minimum course requirements; in such a case, the required course must be successfully completed (grade of C- or higher), and then a higher-level, comparable course must be used to meet that particular requirement.

AP credit policy: must appear on official college transcripts and be equivalent to the appropriate college-level coursework.

Course completion deadline: prerequisites must be completed by the end of the spring term prior to fall matriculation.

Standardized examinations: Graduate Record Exam (GRE®), general test, is required (no minimum score) and is due at the school by October 1.

Additional requirements and considerations

Evaluation of written application (including veterinary/research experience)

Supplemental application

Letters of recommendation (3 submitted through VMCAS; 1 must be completed by a veterinarian)

Interview (by invitation on a competitive basis)

Summary of Admission Procedure

Timetable
> VMCAS application deadline: Friday, October 1, 2010 12:00 PM (noon) Eastern Time
> Date interviews are held: January and February
> Date acceptances mailed: February
> First-year classes begin: early July

Deposit (to hold place in class): $500.00.

Deferments: requests are considered on an individual basis.

Evaluation criteria
> Grades
> Quality of academic program
> Test scores
> Animal/veterinary experience
> Interview
> References (3 required, one by a veterinarian)
> Application (includes personal statement)

2009–2010 admissions summary

	Number of Applicants	Number of New Entrants
Resident	67	42*
Nonresident	763	38*
Total:	824*	80*

*Includes students admitted through the Early Entry Program

Expenses for the 2009–2010 Academic Year

Tuition and fees
Resident	$14,087.00
Nonresident	$32,828.00

Dual-Degree Programs

Combined DVM–graduate degree programs are available.

University of Missouri

Office of Academic Affairs
College of Veterinary Medicine
W203 Veterinary Medicine Building
University of Missouri-Columbia
Columbia MO 65211
Telephone: (573) 884-6435
Email: seayk@missouri.edu
www.missouri.edu

The University of Missouri is located among rolling forested hills north of the famous Lake of the Ozarks. Columbia is noted for its high quality of life and low cost of living and is consistently rated among the best cities to live in by Money Magazine. The city abounds with walking trails, 3,000 acres of state park lands, federal forests, and wildlife refuges. Columbia is located between Kansas City and St. Louis—cities that have major-league sports teams and other big-city recreational amenities. Columbia itself offers Big 12 Conference football, basketball, baseball and other sports. It boasts a 65,000-seat stadium, several 18-hole golf courses, and other indoor and outdoor recreation facilities. Our location near a metropolitan area provides a strong primary and referral small animal case load. Columbia's proximity to rural central Missouri results in an exceptional food animal and equine case load.

MU, a major research university with 30,000 students, consists of 19 schools and colleges located on a 1,335-acre campus. The College of Veterinary Medicine is noted for its unique curriculum that gives students 2 years of undiluted clinical experience before graduation as opposed to the traditional 1–1½ years. Students benefit from exposure to specialty medical areas such as clinical cardi-ology, neurology, orthopedics, ophthalmology, and oncology. Students also gain experience with advanced equipment such as a linear accelerator for treatment of cancer, MRI, state-of-the-art ultrasonography, extensive endoscopy equipment, cold lasers, a surgery room C-arm for radiography during surgical procedures, and others. MU is unique in having a medical school, nursing school, school of health related professions, state cancer research center, the life sciences center, the second largest research animal diagnostic laboratory in the world and department of animal science on the same campus, thus enhancing teaching, research, and clinical services.

Application Information

For specific application information (availability, deadlines, fees, and VMCAS participation), please refer to the contact information listed above.

Residency implications: first priority is given to Missouri residents; second priority is given to nonresidents. U.S. citizenship or permanent residency is required.

Prerequisites for Admission

Course requirements and semester hours

English or communication	6
College algebra or more advanced mathematics	3
Physics	5
Biological science	10
Social sciences or humanities	10
Biochemistry (Organic Chemistry pre-req.)	3
Minimum credit hours	**60**

Required undergraduate GPA: Applicants must have a cumulative GPA of 3.00 or more on a 4.00 scale. The most recent entering class had a mean GPA of 3.70 at the time of acceptance.

AP credit policy: must appear on official college transcript and be equivalent to the appropriate college-level coursework.

Course completion deadline: prerequisite courses must be completed by the end of the winter semester or spring quarter of the year of entry.

Standardized examinations: The Medical College Admission Test (MCAT) or the Graduate Record Examination (GRE®) general test is required. Test scores older than 3 years will not be accepted.

Additional requirements and considerations

    Animal/veterinary experience
    Recommendations/evaluations (3 required)
      Employer
      Academic advisors/faculty member
      Veterinarians
    Extracurricular and/or community service activities
    Essays
      Animal experience
      Explanation of choice of veterinary medicine as a profession
    Employment history

Summary of Admission Procedure

Timetable

    VMCAS application deadline: Friday, October 1, 2010 12:00 PM
      (noon) Eastern Time
    Direct application and supplemental application deadline: November 1

Date interviews are held: February–March (late December–early
    January for non-residents)
Date acceptances mailed: mid-April
School begins: late August

Deposit (to hold place in class): $100.00 for residents; $500.00 for nonresidents.

Deferments: each is considered individually by the admissions committee.

Evaluation criteria

The admission process consists of a preliminary file review of all applicants. Personal interviews are subsequently granted to all qualified Missouri residents and 175 to 200 nonresidents.

	% weight
Grades	35
Test scores	5
Interview score including:	60
Animal/veterinary experience	
Interpersonal skills	
Work ethic	
Leadership in college and community	
Life experiences and diversity	

2009–2010 admissions summary

	Number of Applicants	Number of New Entrants
Resident	139	66
Nonresident	569	44
Total:	708	110

Expenses for the 2009–2010 Academic Year

Tuition and fees

Resident	$17,780.00
Nonresident	$33,496.00

Dual-Degree Programs

Combined DVM–graduate degree programs are available.

Early Admission Program

The Pre-veterinary Medicine and AgScholars Programs guarantee acceptance into the professional program upon satisfactory completion of the undergraduate requirements. Eligibility requires a high-school senior or University of

Missouri freshman to have a composite ACT score of at least 30 and 27 respectively, or an equivalent SAT score. Eligible applicants will be interviewed, and a satisfactory score must be achieved to become a Scholar. Selected veterinary medical faculty will be assigned as mentors. Scholars receive priority consideration for part-time employment in the college. Further information may be obtained by contacting the Office of Academic Affairs.

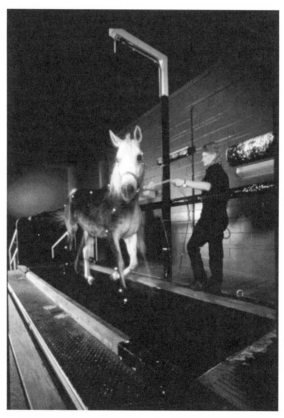

A lame horse is evaluated on a treadmill at the Equine Hospital at the University of Missouri's College of Veterinary Medicine.

North Carolina State University

Student Services Office
College of Veterinary Medicine
North Carolina State University
4700 Hillsborough Street, Box 8401
Raleigh NC 27606
Telephone: (919) 513-6262
Email: cvm_dvm@ncsu.edu
www.cvm.ncsu.edu

The North Carolina State University College of Veterinary Medicine is located on a 182-acre site in Raleigh, the state capital, which has a population of more than 300,000. The sandy shores of North Carolina's beautiful coastline are a short ride to the east, and the Great Smoky Mountains are to the west. The climate includes mild winters and warm summers.

The College of Veterinary Medicine opened in the fall of 1981 and occupies more than 260,000 square feet, including a teaching hospital, classrooms, animal wards, research and teaching laboratories, and an audiovisual area. The college has 120 faculty members and a capacity for 312 veterinary medical students with training for interns, residents, and graduate students.

Construction started fall 2002 on the Centennial Biomedical Campus, which will be anchored by the College of Veterinary Medicine. An extension of the original NCSU Centennial Campus concept, the Centennial Biomedical Campus will house approximately 32 building sites. It will include an additional 1.6 million square feet of space over the next 25 years, resulting in a five-fold expansion of the current college and teaching hospital. The two-year construction of the Randall B. Terry, Jr. Companion Animal Veterinary Medical Center is underway at the College of Veterinary Medicine. When completed in late 2010, the Terry Center is expected to be the national model for excellence in companion animal medicine. The Terry Center will offer cutting-edge technologies for imaging, cardiac care, cancer treatments, internal medicine, and surgery; will more than double the size of the current companion animal hospital; and will help accommodate the more than 20,000 cases referred to the CVM each year.

The Centennial Biomedical Campus will emphasize partnerships that work to bring academia, government and industry together. The focus of this campus is on biomedical applications, both to animals and humans. It will provide opportunities for industry and government researchers, entrepreneurs, clinical trial companies, as well as collaborations with other universities to work side by side with faculty and students at the College of Veterinary Medicine.

Application Information

For specific application information (availability, deadlines, fees, and VMCAS participation), please refer to the contact information listed above.

Residency implications: priority is given to North Carolina residents. There are approximately 18 nonresident positions.

Prerequisites for Admission

Course requirements and semester hours

Any combination of English composition I, English composition II, public speaking, or communication	6
College calculus	3
Introduction to statistics	3
General physics I, II (with laboratory)	8
General chemistry I, II (with laboratory)	8
Organic chemistry I, II (with laboratory)	8
General biology (with laboratory)	4
Principles of genetics	4
General microbiology (with laboratory)	4
Biochemistry	3
Social sciences and humanities	6
Animal nutrition	3

AP credit policy: must appear on official college transcripts and be equivalent to the appropriate college-level coursework.

Course completion deadline: only 2 courses may be pending completion in the spring semester, and both must be completed (with transcript evidence) by the end of the spring semester prior to matriculation. Pending courses (including correspondence courses) may not be completed in the summer session immediately preceding matriculation.

Standardized examinations: Graduate Record Examination (GRE®), general test, is required. The scores must be received by the October 1 application deadline.

Additional requirements and considerations

Animal/veterinary knowledge, experience, motivation, and maturity
Personal statement
Recommendations/evaluations (3 required; at least 2 from veterinarians/scientists with whom applicant has worked is highly recommended)
Extracurricular activities

Summary of Admission Procedure

Timetable
> VMCAS application deadline: Friday, October 1, 2010 12:00 PM (noon)
>   Eastern Time (VMCAS and NC State supplemental)
> Date acceptances mailed: no later than April 1
> School begins: August

Deposit (to hold place in class): $250.00.

Deferments: are considered for 1 year only, subject to Admissions Committee approval.

Evaluation criteria
Selection for admission is a 2-phase process:

Phase 1—Objective criteria:
> Required course GPA: 3.3 Resident, 3.4 Nonresident
> Cumulative GPA: 3.0 Resident, 3.4 Nonresident
> GPA in last 45+ credits attempted: 3.3 Resident, 3.4 Nonresident
> GRE test score
> Supplemental Application

Phase 2—Subjective score:
> Applicant folder review by admissions committee

2009–2010 admissions summary

	Number of Applicants	Number of New Entrants*
Resident	210	62
Nonresident	522	18
Total:	732	80

* Estimated

Expenses for the 2009–2010 Academic Year

Tuition and fees
Resident	$10,937.00
Nonresident	$33,700.00

Dual Degree Programs

Combined DVM–graduate degree programs are available.

Early Admission Program

Two special admissions options are available: (1) for North Carolina residents focusing on swine, poultry, or food animal medicine in concert with the College of Agriculture and Life Sciences, and (2) for students focusing on laboratory animal medicine in concert with the College of Agriculture at North Carolina A&T State University.

The Ohio State University

Office of Student Affairs
College of Veterinary Medicine
Suite 127 Veterinary Medicine Academic Building
1900 Coffey Road
The Ohio State University
Columbus OH 43210-1089
Telephone: (614) 292-8831
Fax: (614) 292-6989
Email: students@cvm.osu.edu
www.vet.ohio-state.edu

Ohio State University is located in Columbus, the capital of Ohio. Columbus is a congregation of cities and villages with a sense of history and a friendly atmosphere. The third-ranking center of scientific and technological research and data dissemination in the United States, the city offers fine arts, restaurants, sports, architecture, nature, community festivals, churches, and other areas of interest.

The Ohio State University is one of the nation's leading academic centers, with a sprawling campus straddling the Olentangy River. The campus consists of thousands of acres, hundreds of buildings, more than 15,000 faculty and staff, and more than 54,000 students. The veterinary college is the third-oldest in the United States and is one of the largest veterinary colleges in North America. The patient load is one of the highest in the country, and farmlands can be accessed 10 miles from campus. The faculty members have diverse academic and research activities, and 85 percent of the clinical teaching faculty are board certified. The academic curriculum is a 4-year program that blends some clinical experience into the first 2 years, while the last 2 years are mostly clinical.

Application Information

For specific application information (availability, deadlines, fees, and VMCAS participation), please refer to the contact information listed above.

Residency implications: priority is given to Ohio residents. Ohio State will accept nonresident students.

Prerequisites for Admission

For the humanities and social sciences requirement, students are encouraged to elect the courses required for the bachelor of science curriculum. Courses in communication, journalism, sociology, economics, and animal behavior are strongly recommended. Elective courses are at the student's discretion, after consultation with an advisor. However, highly recommended electives include embryology, histology, cell biology, immunology, anatomy, physiology, and animal science including nutrition

Students enrolled in the preveterinary medicine curriculum are encouraged to take electives that will provide a well-rounded education in addition to those biological sciences preparatory to the veterinary medical curriculum.

Course requirements and quarter hours

English	5
General chemistry (with laboratory)*	15
Organic chemistry*	6
Biochemistry*	5
Biology*	10
Genetics*	5
Microbiology (with laboratory)*	5
Mathematics (algebra and trigonometry)	5
General physics (with laboratory)*	10
Humanities and social sciences	20
Electives	10

* Must have been completed within the 10 years preceding the application deadline.

Graduate students must have a letter from their advisor releasing them from their graduate program if accepted into the veterinary medicine program.

Required undergraduate GPA: the required GPA for an interview is 3.0 on a 4.0 scale. The most recent entering class had a mean overall GPA of 3.72 and a science GPA of 3.68. Science and math GPA are evaluated as well as last 45 semester or quarter hours.

AP credit policy: AP credit given if course is listed on official transcript.

Course completion deadline: all but one prerequisite course must be completed by the end of the fall semester or quarter coinciding with submission of the application. The final remaining prerequisite course must be completed at the end of the following term (spring semester or winter quarter). Failure to satisfactorily complete all prerequisites with a grade of C or better will result in automatic loss of a candidate's seat in the class.

Standardized examinations: Scores from one of the following standardized examinations must be submitted at the time of application:

> *Graduate Record Examination (GRE®):* minimum acceptable score 1000 total of all three subtests.
> *Medical College Admission Test (MCAT):* minimum acceptable score 25 total; score O-T on essay portion (new MCAT).

Scores must not be older than five years prior to the application year. The most recent acceptable date for taking the examination is September 30 of the application year.

Additional requirements and considerations
> Academic background/difficulty
> Minimum of 80 hours work with a single veterinarian (volunteer or paid)
> Interpersonal skills/communication skills
> Motivation/commitment/initiative/innovative
> Animal handling experience
> Veterinary experience
> Knowledge and understanding of the profession
> Letters of recommendation (2 must be from veterinarians). Evaluators may not be relatives.
> Written communication
> Integrity/leadership/adversity

Summary of Admission Procedure

Timetable
> VMCAS application deadline: Friday, October 1, 2010 12:00 PM (noon) Eastern Time
> Date interviews are held: December–January
> Date acceptances mailed: December–March
> School begins: late September

Deposit (to hold place in class): $25.00 for residents; $300.00 (non-refundable fee) for contract and nonresident applicants.

Deferments: not considered.

Evaluation criteria

	% *weight*
Objective score	45
Subjective score	55

* Preferred applicants are interviewed and evaluated by members of the Admissions Committee. The academic interview covers subjective areas such as communication/interpersonal skills, motivation/initiative/innovation, animal handling experience, veterinary experience, involvement in social and community activities, motivation and commitment to veterinary medicine, comprehension of veterinary medicine, knowledge of and/or exposure to animals,. Those applicants given the highest overall evaluation are selected for the entering class.

2009–2010 admissions summary

	Number of Applicants	Number of New Entrants
Resident	243	100
Nonresident	551	40
Total:	794	140

Expenses for the 2008–2009 Academic Year

Estimated tuition and fees (subject to change)

Resident	$23,598.00
Nonresident*	$55,440.00

* For tuition purposes, **nonresident students can apply for residency after completing their first year at Ohio State.**

Dual-Degree Programs

Combined DVM–graduate degree programs are available.

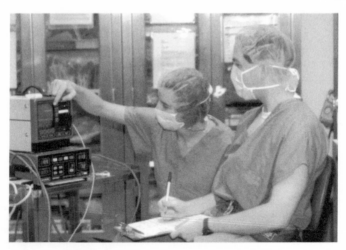

Veterinary students monitor the vital signs of a patient during surgery at the North Carolina State University Veterinary Teaching Hospital. Photo courtesy of North Carolina State University College of Veterinary Medicine.

Oklahoma State University

Office of Admissions
112 McElroy Hall
Center for Veterinary Health Sciences
College of Veterinary Medicine
Oklahoma State University
Stillwater OK 74078-2003
Telephone: (405) 744-6961
Fax: (405) 744-0356
Email: anna.teague@okstate.edu
www.cvhs.okstate.edu

Oklahoma State University is located in Stillwater, which has a population of about 47,000. Stillwater is in north central Oklahoma about 65 miles from Oklahoma City and 69 miles from Tulsa. The campus is exceptionally beautiful, with modified Georgian-style architecture in the new buildings. It encompasses 840 acres and more than 60 major academic buildings.

Three major buildings form the veterinary medicine complex. The oldest, McElroy Hall, houses the William E. Brock Memorial Library and Learning Center, as well as new classrooms and laboratories. The Boren Veterinary Medical Teaching Hospital provides modern facilities for both academic and clinical instruction. Completing the triad is the Oklahoma Animal Disease Diagnostic Laboratory, which provides teaching resources for students in the professional curriculum and diagnostic services to Oklahoma agriculture and industry. The College of Veterinary Medicine is fully accredited by the American Veterinary Medical Association. Faculty members in the 3 academic departments share responsibility for the curriculum. These departments are Veterinary Clinical Sciences, Veterinary Pathobiology, and Physiological Sciences.

Application Information

For specific application information (availability, deadlines, fees, and VMCAS participation), please refer to the contact information listed above.

Residency implications: priority is given to Oklahoma residents. Nonresidents may apply, and Oklahoma State could admit up to 2 contract students from New Jersey and up to 22 first-time nonresident students (including any contract students from Arkansas or Delaware).

Prerequisites for Admission

Course requirements and semester hours
    English composition   6

English elective	3
General chemistry (with laboratory)	8–10
Organic chemistry (with laboratory)	8
Biochemistry	3
Physics	8
Mathematics	3
Zoology (with laboratory)	4
Animal nutrition	3
Biological science	3
Microbiology (with laboratory)	4–5
Genetics (laboratory recommended)	3–4
Humanities or social sciences	6
Electives (science or business)	2

Required undergraduate GPA: a minimum GPA of 2.80 on a 4.00 scale is required in prerequisite courses. The mean cumulative GPA of the 2009 entering class was 3.52.

AP credit policy: AP credit accepted if documented on college transcript.

Course completion deadline: prerequisite courses must be completed by the end of the spring semester just prior to matriculation.

Standardized examinations: Graduate Record Examination (GRE®), general test and biology subject test, is required. Earliest acceptable test date is June 2005. The class of 2013 had mean scores of 477 verbal, 628quantitative, and 560 biology.

Additional requirements and considerations
    Evidence of motivation over an extended period of time
    Animal/veterinary work experience
    Amount of undergraduate education completed
    Recommendations/evaluations (3 required)
        Veterinarian (required)
        Academic advisor, preferred
        Employer
    Demonstrated leadership and interpersonal skills

All science courses must have been taken within 8 years of application (fall 2002 for class entering fall 2011)

Summary of Admission Procedure

Timetable
    VMCAS application deadline: Friday, October 1, 2010 12:00 PM
    (noon) Eastern Time

Date interviews held: February
Date acceptances mailed: March
School begins: mid-August

Deposit (to hold place in class): resident, $100.00; nonresident, $500.00.

Deferments: to complete graduate degree, deferments are considered.

Evaluation criteria
The admission procedure consists of evaluation of both academic and nonacademic criteria. The Admissions Committee considers all factors in the applicant's file, but the following are especially important: academic achievement; familiarity with the profession and sincerity of interest; recommendations; test scores; extracurricular activities; character, personality, and general fitness and commitment for a career in veterinary medicine. The committee selects those applicants considered most capable of excelling as veterinary medical students and who possess the greatest potential for success in the veterinary medical profession.

2009–2010 admissions summary

	Number of Applicants	Number of New Entrants
Resident	116	58
Nonresident	336	24
Total:	452	82

Expenses for the 2008–2009 Academic Year

Tuition and fees
Resident	$14,300.00
Nonresident	$31,600.00

Dual-Degree Programs

Combined DVM–graduate and MBA/DVM degree programs are available.

Early Admissions

The Early Admit Program offers an admissions avenue for those senior high school students with exceptional academic performance, maturity and commitment to veterinary medicine and Oklahoma State University. Applicants must have an ACT score of 27 or higher and complete a successful interview during the fall semester of their freshman undergraduate year. Further information may be obtained by contacting the Office of Admissions and Recruiting at the address noted in previous sections.

Oregon State University

Office of the Dean
Attention: Admissions
College of Veterinary Medicine
Oregon State University
200 Magruder Hall
Corvallis, OR 97331-4801
Telephone: (541) 737-2098
Fax: (541) 737-4245
Email: cvmadmissions@oregonstate.edu
www.oregonstate.edu/vetmed

Oregon State University (OSU) is one of only two universities in the United States to hold the Land Grant, Sea Grant, Sun Grant, and Space Grant designations, and is one of only four doctoral-granting universities in the Pacific Northwest to hold the designation of "very high research" by the Carnegie Foundation. OSU is located in Corvallis, a community of 54,000 people situated in the Willamette Valley between Portland and Eugene. Ocean beaches, lakes, rivers, forests, high desert, and the rugged Cascade and Coast Ranges are all within a 100-mile drive of Corvallis. Life in Corvallis includes lectures, concerts, films, and exhibits through the university. In the heart of the agriculturally-rich Willamette River Valley, Corvallis enjoys colorful and crisp autumns, mild and rainy winters, flowering springs, and warm, dry summers.

The first class of veterinary students entered Oregon State University in the fall of 1979, coinciding with the opening of the university's large animal hospital. Starting with the class entering in 2003, the College has offered a fully accredited, four-year program in Corvallis. The OSU College of Veterinary Medicine (CVM) supports small animal, equine, camelid, and food animal medicine and surgery as well as diagnostic and pathology services. The College opened a state-of-the-art small animal clinic in 2005 and renovation and expansion of the large animal facilities were completed in 2008. The College faculty has recently grown with faculty numbers nearly doubling in the last four years. The small class size of 56 students helps to provide them with an excellent veterinary education and the opportunity to have close interaction with faculty.

Application Information

For specific application information (availability, deadlines, fees, and VMCAS participation), please refer to the contact information listed above.

Residency implications: Oregon residents and WICHE-sponsored students are eligible for resident fees. Up to 20 students are accepted as nonresidents including applicants from WICHE states.

Prerequisites for Admission

Science course requirements

General biology	A course sequence of biology (2 semesters or 3 quarters).
Biological sciences	A minimum of at least 4 additional semester or 6 additional quarter credits of upper-division biological science courses with at least one laboratory.
Physics	A course sequence in physics for science majors (2 semesters or 3 quarters).
General chemistry	A course sequence of inorganic chemistry with laboratories (2 semesters or 3 quarters).
Organic chemistry	A course sequence of organic chemistry sufficient to meet requirements for upper-division biochemistry (1-2 semesters or 2-3 quarters).
Biochemistry	A minimum of 1 semester or 2 quarters of upper-division biochemistry; a complete course sequence is preferred.
Animal nutrition	A course in general animal nutrition that includes monogastric and ruminant nutrition (at least 2 semester or 3 quarter credits).
Genetics	A course in general genetics that includes both Mendelian and molecular genetics (at least 3 semester or 4 quarter credits).
Mathematics	A course in calculus (at least 2 semester or 3 quarter credits).
Physiology	A course in animal or human physiology (at least 2 semester or 3 quarter credits).
Statistics	A course(s) in statistics (at least 3 semester or 4 quarter credits).

General education course requirements

English	At least 4 semester or 6 quarter credits of English writing (e.g., English composition, technical writing).
Public speaking	At least 2 semester or 3 quarter credits of public speaking.

| Humanities/social sciences | At least 8 semester or 12 quarter credits of humanities or social science courses. |

These requirements will be considered met if the applicant has a bachelor's degree by July 1 of the year in which they are accepted into the program.

All prerequisite courses taken after August 2004 must be graded on an A–F scale and not taken as pass/fail. Any grade below C– in a prerequisite course is considered unsatisfactory and the course cannot be accepted to fulfill a requirement. Applicants can fulfill the requirement by repeating the same course or by substituting a higher-level course in the same field as that of the required course. A student who attends an institution that does not provide traditional grades will be evaluated on an individual basis. In addition to the prerequisite courses, applicants are encouraged to take elective courses to better prepare them for the veterinary curriculum and profession. Suggested electives include courses in animal science, business, embryology and microbiology.

Required undergraduate GPA: A minimum GPA is not required, however students with a GPA below 3.20 are rarely admitted to the program. The average cumulative GPA of admitted students is approximately 3.60.

AP credit policy: Advanced Placement (AP) and College Level Examination Program (CLEP) exam credit for lower-division prerequisite courses is accepted; credit must be reflected on the official ETS College Board score report or on an official college transcript.

Course completion deadline: Students must complete prerequisite courses by July 1 prior to matriculation. Complete and final official academic transcripts for all accepted applicants must be received by OSU CVM by August 1 prior to matriculation. It is the applicant's responsibility to verify receipt of these materials.

Standardized examinations: Graduate Record Examination (GRE®), general test, is required. The GRE must be taken within a five-year period prior to applying to veterinary school. Test scores must be submitted by the application deadline, October 1, 2010. It is the applicant's responsibility to verify receipt of these materials.

Additional requirements and considerations
    Quality and rigor of academic preparation
    Evidence of desirable skills, knowledge, attitude, and aptitude
    Animal/veterinary knowledge and experience
    Recommendations/evaluations (three required, at least one by a
        veterinarian)
    Interview (Oregon residents only)

Summary of Admission Procedure

Timetable

> VMCAS application deadline: Friday, October 1, 2010 12:00 PM
>   (noon) Eastern Time
> Supplemental application receipt deadline: October 1, 2010
> Date interviews are held: February
> Date acceptances mailed: February–March
> School begins: late September

Deposit (to hold place in class): $50.00. Deferments: considered on an individual basis.

Evaluation criteria

Major criteria upon which applicants are selected include likelihood of academic success in the program, demonstration of qualities deemed valuable in a veterinarian, exposure to and an understanding of the veterinary profession, and diversity. Academic criteria include undergraduate and graduate grades, quantity and quality of upper-division science courses, performance in prerequisite courses, academic credit load, GRE scores, and work and/or family demands during school. Nonacademic factors considered are interpersonal skills, communication skills, integrity, maturity, motivation, civic and community-mindedness, diversity of interests and activities, leadership in student and/or community organizations, scientific inquisitiveness and analytical skills. Academic and nonacademic factors are determined by evaluation of the VMCAS application, supplemental application, letters of evaluation and interview (Oregon residents only).

Oregon State University does not discriminate on the basis of race, color, gender, national origin, religion, sexual orientation, age, marital status, disability, or veteran status.

2008–2009 admissions summary

	Number of Applicants	Number of New Entrants
Resident	97	40
Contract (WICHE)*	149	1
Nonresident	270	15
Total:	516	56

* For further information, see the listing of contracting states and provinces.

Expenses for the 2009–2010 Academic Year

Tuition and fees

> Resident (approximate) $18,627.81

Nonresident
   Contract* $18,627.81
   Other nonresident (approximate) $35,952.81

* For further information, see the listing of contracting states and provinces.

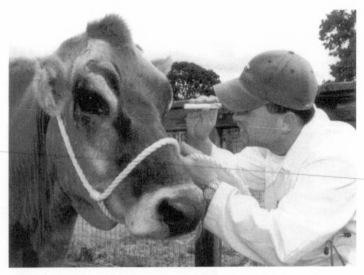

Up close and personal: with practice, students develop examination skills to deal with all sorts of patients. Photo courtesy of Oregon State University College of Veterinary Medicine.

University of Pennsylvania

Admissions Office
School of Veterinary Medicine
3800 Spruce Street University of Pennsylvania
Philadelphia PA 19104-6044
Telephone: (215) 898-5434
Fax: (215) 573-8819
Email: admissions@vet.upenn.edu
www.vet.upenn.edu

The University of Pennsylvania is located in West Philadelphia. Philadelphia is a city with a strong cultural heritage. Independence National Park includes 1 square mile of historic Philadelphia next to the Delaware River. Included are Independence Hall, the Liberty Bell, and many fine examples of colonial architecture. Philadelphia also offers theaters, museums, sports, and outdoor recreation. The Philadelphia Zoo, first in the nation, houses more than 1,600 mammals, birds, reptiles, and amphibians. The School of Veterinary Medicine enjoys a close relationship with the zoo.

The School of Veterinary Medicine was founded in 1884 and includes a hospital for small animals, classrooms, and research facilities in the city. The large-animal hospital and research facilities are located at the New Bolton Center, an 800-acre farm 40 miles west of Philadelphia. The first 2 years are spent on the main campus. Part of the third year may be spent at the New Bolton Center, and the fourth year is spent in rotation and on electives at varying campus locations. Off-campus electives are frequently permitted.

Application Information

For specific application information (availability, deadlines, fees, and VMCAS participation), please refer to the contact information listed above.

Residency implications: priority is given to Pennsylvania residents. The number of nonresident places is usually 78, including international applicants.

Prerequisites for Admission

At least 3 English credits must be in composition; biology courses must provide background in genetics. Organic chemistry must cover aliphatic and aromatic compounds to fulfill the requirement.

Course requirements and semester hours

English (including composition)	6
Physics (with laboratory)	8
Chemistry (with at least 1 laboratory)	
General	8
Organic	4
Biology or zoology (3 courses)	9
Social sciences or humanities	6
Calculus and math statistics (or biostats)	6
Electives	43

(Although not required, biochemistry is strongly recommended.)

Required undergraduate GPA: no specific GPA. Applicants are evaluated comparatively. The mean cumulative GPA of the class admitted in 2009 was 3.61.

AP credit policy: must appear on official college transcripts and count toward degree.

Course completion deadline: prerequisite courses must be completed by the end of the summer term of the year in which admission is sought.

Standardized examinations: Graduate Record Examination (GRE®), general test, is required; the GRE Code for Pennvet is 2775. Test scores should be received no later than December 1. The class admitted in 2009 had an average of 578 on the verbal subtest and 710 on the quantitative subtest.

Additional requirements and considerations

Animal/veterinary work experience: experience working with animals, direct veterinary work, or research experience is desired. No minimum time limit. Experience should be sufficient to convince the admissions committee of motivation, interest, and understanding.

Recommendations/evaluations: 3 required, one from an academic science source; and one from a veterinarian. The third is the choice of the applicant.

Extracurricular/community service activities: additional activities in this category can provide information important to the admissions committee.

Leadership: evidence of leadership abilities is desirable.

Summary of Admission Procedure

Timetable
> VMCAS application deadline: Friday, October 1, 2010 12:00 PM
> (noon) Eastern Time
> Supplemental application and fee deadline: October 1
> Date interviews are held: Fridays from early January until completion
> Date acceptances mailed: within 14 days after interview
> School begins: early September

Deposit (to hold place in class): $500.00. Deferments: are considered on an individual basis.

Evaluation criteria
The seats are filled through a 2-part admission procedure, which includes a file review and personal interviews.
> Grades
> Test scores
> Animal/veterinary experience
> Interview
> References
> Essay
> English skills (TOEFL)

File review: files are reviewed in January by pairs of members of the admissions committee (including an alumni member), and decisions are made on whether or not to offer an interview.

Personal interviews: interviews are held on Fridays from early January until the class is filled. The number of interviews granted equals 1½ to 2 times the number of seats available.

Two personal interviews are conducted: a formal interview with 2 faculty members (including an alumni member) of the committee, and an informal interview with student committee members. Although students do not vote on acceptance, they have a significant part in the meeting following interviews.

2009–2010 admissions summary

	Number of Applicants	Number of New Entrants
Resident	242	65
Nonresident	1,127	57
Total:	1,369	122

Expenses for the 2009–2010 Academic Year

Tuition and fees
Resident $33,814.00
Nonresident $42,398.00

Dual-Degree Programs

Combined VMD–graduate degree programs are available.

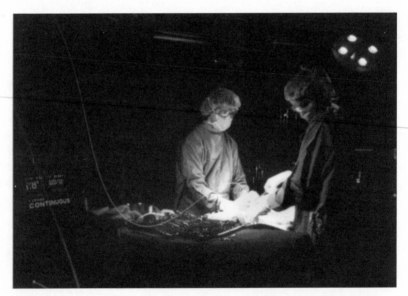

Veterinarians at Oklahoma State University's College of Veterinary Medicine perform laser surgery as part of their investigation of the medical application of lasers. Photo courtesy of the College of Veterinary Medicine, Oklahoma State University.

Purdue University

Admissions and Student Services Office
School of Veterinary Medicine
Lynn Hall, 1185
625 Harrison Street
Purdue University
West Lafayette IN 47907-2026
Telephone: (765) 494-7893 or (800) 213-2859 (long distance)
Email: vetadmissions@purdue.edu
www.vet.purdue.edu/admissions

Purdue University is located in one of the largest metropolitan centers in northwestern Indiana. Greater Lafayette occupies a site on the Wabash River 65 miles northwest of Indianapolis and 126 miles southeast of Chicago. The combined population of the twin cities, Lafayette and West Lafayette, exceeds 64,000. The community offers an art museum, historical museum, 1,600 acres of public parks, and more than 60 churches of all major denominations.

Purdue ranks among the 25 largest colleges and universities in the nation. Students represent all 50 states and many foreign countries. Diversity and opportunity are goals that the School of Veterinary Medicine maintains in the selection of each year's entering class. The School of Veterinary Medicine has assumed a leading position nationally and internationally in veterinary education. To better prepare individuals for veterinary medical careers in the twenty-first century, our curriculum emphasizes the veterinary team approach using new and innovative strategies.

Application Information

For specific application information (availability, deadlines, fees, and VMCAS participation), please refer to the contact information listed above.

Residency implications: priority is given to Indiana residents. Approximately one-third of the class will be nonresident students in a total class of 70. Applicants from all states will be considered. Purdue has no contract positions. International applicants will be considered provided both the academic and financial criteria can be met.

Prerequisites for Admission

The course requirements outlined below are considered the bare minimum prerequisite courses to be completed. No less than a grade of C must be received in each required course in order to be considered eligible for admission. In the electives category, humanities include languages, cognitive sciences, and social sciences. Other courses are highly recommended and can be found on our web site.

Course requirements and number of semesters

Inorganic chemistry with lab	2
Organic chemistry with lab	2
Biochemistry	1
Biology with lab (diversity, developmental, cell structure)	2
Genetics with lab	1
Microbiology (general or medical) with lab	1
Nutrition (animal)	1
Physics with lab	2
Calculus	1
Statistics	1
English composition	1
Communication (interpersonal, persuasion or speech)	1
Careers in Veterinary Medicine (if available)	1
Humanities (foreign languages, cognitive sciences, and social sciences)	3

Note: Complete course sequences should be followed rather than focusing on credit hours.

Required undergraduate GPA: the mean cumulative GPA of the 2009 entering class was 3.56 on a 4.00 scale. The minimum overall GPA required for consideration is 3.00 on a 4.00 scale for nonresident applicants and 2.75 on a 4.00 scale for resident applicants.

AP credit policy: must appear on official college transcripts by subject area and be equivalent to the appropriate college-level coursework.

Course completion deadline: minimum prerequisite courses must be completed by the end of the spring term prior to matriculation.

Standardized examinations: Graduate Record Examination (GRE®), general test, is required. Test scores must be received no later than October 1 of the year of application. Use the Grad School GRE code of 1631.

Additional requirements and considerations
> Animal/veterinary/research experience
> Amount of college education
> Recommendations/evaluations (3 required)
>> Academic advisor/faculty member
>> Employer
>> Veterinarian
> Essay
> Employment record
> Extracurricular college experience

Summary of Admission Procedure

Timetable
> VMCAS application deadline: Friday, October 1, 2010 12:00 PM
> > (noon) Eastern Time
> Date interviews are held: February
> Date acceptances mailed: March
> School begins: late August

Deposit (to hold place in class): $250.00 for residents; $1,000.00 for non-residents.

Deferments: request for deferments will be considered on a case-by-case basis.

Evaluation criteria
The admission process consists of:
> A preliminary review based upon grade point indices, test scores, and
> > prerequisite course completion
> An in-depth review of selected applicants
> A personal interview by invitation

	% weight
Grades, test scores, overall academic performance (including honors courses, study abroad)	55
Animal, veterinary, research, and general work experiences, extracurricular activities, essay, overall presentation of application materials, references, and interview	45

2009–2010 admissions summary

	Number of Applicants	Number of New Entrants
Resident	110	39
Nonresident	551	30
International	1	1
Total:	661	70

Expenses for the 2009–2010 Academic Year

Tuition and fees
Resident	$17,018.00
Nonresident	$40,286.00

Dual-Degree Programs
Combined DVM–graduate degree programs are available.

Early Admission Program

The Veterinary Scholars Program provides an opportunity for early admission into the professional program by accepting high-school seniors who

1. rank in the top 10 percent of their graduating class;
2. have attained a combined SAT score equal to or greater than 1950 or composite ACT score equal to or greater than 28;
3. were admitted to Purdue University and committed to a major in animal sciences, biochemistry, or biological sciences programs; and
4. demonstrate a background of work experience with animals and veterinarians.

Students admitted to the program must complete all preveterinary prerequisite coursework, obtain a bachelor's degree with stipulated grade point averages for each year of undergraduate study, and submit scores from the GRE® (Graduate Record Exam), general test, during their senior year.

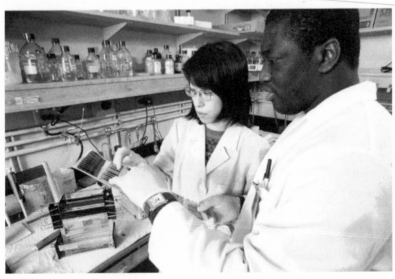

Many veterinary medical students choose a career in research rather than a clinical practice. Photo by Vincent P. Walter, courtesy of Purdue University.

University of Tennessee

Admissions Office
College of Veterinary Medicine
2407 River Drive
Room A-104-C
Knoxville TN 37996-4550
Telephone: (865) 974-7354
Email: dshepherd@utk.edu
www.vet.utk.edu

The University of Tennessee's College of Veterinary Medicine is located in Knoxville, a city of 185,000 situated in the Appalachian foothills of east central Tennessee. Only 45 minutes from the Great Smoky Mountains National Park and 3 hours from both Nashville and Atlanta, Knoxville offers many recreational and cultural opportunities, including a symphony orchestra, an opera company, and several fine theaters. The climate in Knoxville is moderate with distinct seasons.

The 550-acre Knoxville campus of the University of Tennessee has about 20,400 undergraduate and 6,000 graduate students. The modern Clyde M. York Veterinary Medicine Building, housing the teaching and research facilities, the W.W. Armistead Veterinary Teaching Hospital, and Agriculture-Veterinary Medicine Library, faces the Tennessee River on the university's Agricultural Campus.

The curriculum of the College of Veterinary Medicine is a 9-semester, 4-year program. Development of a strong basic science education is emphasized in the first year. The second and third years emphasize the study of diseases, their causes, diagnosis, treatment, and prevention. Innovative features of the first three years of the curriculum include 6 weeks of student-centered small-group applied-learning exercises in semesters 1–5; 3 weeks of dedicated clinical experiences in the veterinary teaching hospital in semesters 3–5; and elective course opportunities in semesters 4–9 that allow students to focus on specific educational/ career goals. In the fourth year (final 3 semesters), students participate exclusively in clinical rotations (27 weeks of core rotations and 17 weeks of elective rotations) in the W.W. Armistead Veterinary Teaching Hospital and in required off-campus externships. The college has unique programs in zoo, avian, and exotic animal medicine and surgery, cancer diagnosis and therapy, endoscopy, laser surgery, and rehabilitation/physical therapy.

Application Information

For specific application information (availability, deadlines, fees, and VMCAS participation), please refer to the contact information listed above.

Residency implications: priority is given to Tennessee residents. Tennessee has no contractual agreements and does accept nonresident applications.

Prerequisites for Admission

Course requirements and semester hours

General inorganic chemistry (with laboratory)	8
Organic chemistry (with laboratory)	8
General biology/zoology (with laboratory)	8
Cellular/Molecular biology*	3
Genetics	3
Biochemistry (exclusive of laboratory)†	4
Physics (with laboratory)	8
English composition	6
Social sciences/humanities	18

* It is expected that this requirement will be fulfilled by a course in cellular or molecular biology. An upper-division cell or molecular biology course is preferred.

† This should be a complete upper-division course in general cellular and comparative biochemistry. Half of a 2-semester sequence will not satisfy this requirement.

Applicants are strongly encouraged to complete additional biological and physical science courses, especially comparative anatomy, mammalian physiology, microbiology with laboratory, and statistics.

AP credit policy: must appear on official college transcripts and be equivalent to the appropriate college-level coursework.

Required undergraduate GPA: for nonresident applicants, the minimum acceptable cumulative GPA is 3.20 on a 4.00 scale. At time of acceptance, the mean GPA of the class entering in fall of 2009 was 3.60.

Course completion deadline: prerequisite courses must be completed with a grade of C or better by the end of the spring term prior to entry.

Standardized examinations: Graduate Record Exam (GRE®), general test, is required. For applicants planning to matriculate in August 2011, the oldest acceptable GRE scores are from the November 1, 2006, test date.

Additional requirements and considerations

Animal/veterinary work experience
Recommendations/evaluations
Extracurricular and/or community service activities
Leadership skills
Autobiographical essay (personal statement)

Summary of Admission Procedure

Timetable
> VMCAS application deadline: Friday, October 1, 2010 12:00 PM
> > (noon) Eastern Time
> GRE Scores must be received by the College no later than November 15
> Date interviews are held: mid- to late March
> Date acceptances mailed: no later than April 1
> Applicant's response date: April 15
> School begins: late August

Deposit (to hold place in class): none required. Deferments: are considered on a case-by-case basis.

Evaluation criteria
The admission procedure consists of an initial file review followed by an interview of selected applicants.
> Initial academic file review:
> > Grades
> > Test scores
> Interview
> > Animal/veterinary experience
> > Evidence of logical preparation for this career
> > Extracurricular activities/community service
> > Personal interests and qualities
> > References (3-5 required)
> > Essay

2009–2010 admissions summary

	Number of Applicants	Number of New Entrants
Resident	169	60
Nonresident	656	25
Total:	825	85

Expenses for the 2009–2010 Academic Year

Tuition and fees

Resident	$18,366.00
Nonresident	$40,834.00

Parallel Degree Program

The College, in partnership with the College of Education, Health and Human Sciences, offers an option for veterinary students (and graduate veterinarians) to earn the MPH degree with a concentration in Veterinary Public Health. Contact the College of Veterinary Medicine, Dr. John Coy New Jr. at jnew@ utk.edu for additional information.

Texas A & M University

Office of the Dean
Attn: Student Admissions
College of Veterinary Medicine
Texas A & M University
College Station TX 77843-4461
Telephone: (979) 862-1169
www.cvm.tamu.edu

The university is located adjacent to the cities of Bryan and College Station. The two cities have a combined population of about 100,000. The student population at Texas A & M is more than 40,000. The College of Veterinary Medicine is one of the 10 original veterinary teaching institutions that existed in the United States prior to World War II.

The College provides an integrated professional curriculum that prepares graduates with a firm foundation in the basic sciences, a broad comparative medicine knowledge base, and the clinical and personal skills to be leaders in the many career fields of veterinary medicine. Professional students are given the opportunity to gain additional education and training in their personal career paths.

Becoming a veterinarian requires much dedication and diligent study. The veterinary medical student is required to meet a high level of performance. The demands on students' time and effort are considerable, but the rewards and career satisfaction are personal achievements that make significant contributions to our society.

Application Information

For specific application information (availability, deadlines and fees), please refer to the contact information listed above.

Residency implications: Texas has no contractual agreements with other states. Applicants from other states who have outstanding credentials will be considered. Successful candidates who are awarded competitive university-based scholarships may attend at resident tuition rate.

Prerequisites for Admission

The minimum number of college or university credits required for admission into the professional curriculum is 73 semester hours. Applicants must have completed or have in progress approximately 57 credit hours at the time of application. Because there is no specific degree plan associated with pre-veterinary education, students are encouraged to pursue a degree plan that meets individual interests. Students are strongly encouraged to choose courses with the assistance of a knowledgeable counselor at the undergraduate institution or through contact with an academic advisor at the College of Veterinary Medicine, telephone: (979) 862-1169.

Course requirements and semester hours (subject to change)

Life sciences

General biology (with laboratory)	4
*General microbiology (with laboratory)	4
*Genetics	3
*Animal nutrition or feeds and feeding	3
General Animal Science	3

Chemical-physical sciences and mathematics

Inorganic chemistry (with laboratory)	8
Organic chemistry (with laboratory)	8
*Biochemistry I & II(lecture hours only)	5
Calculus or *statistics	3
Physics (with laboratory)	8

Nonscience

Composition and Rhetoric	3
Any Literature course	3
Speech Communications	3
Technical writing	3

* These courses must be taken at a 4-year college or university. These courses may not be taken at community or junior colleges.

Additional credits

In addition to the 61 credit hours recommended above, an applicant must complete a minimum of 12 additional credits. Applicants should keep in mind their degree program, the core curriculum requirements for a baccalaureate degree at Texas A & M University, and their personal career goals in making these choices. Applicants are strongly encouraged to make these choices with a qualified counselor at their institution.

Required undergraduate GPA: the minimum overall GPA required is 2.90 on a 4.00 scale or 3.10 for the last 45 semester credits. The mean of the most recent entering class was 3.64.

AP credit policy: AP credit is accepted as fulfilling selected prerequisites; credit must be reflected on the official undergraduate transcript.

Course completion deadline: required courses must be completed by the end of the spring term prior to entry.

Standardized examinations: Graduate Record Examination (GRE®), general test, is required. The GRE must have been taken within the last five years. The last date to take the GRE (general test) exam is September 30 of the year of application.

Additional requirements and considerations
    Evaluations
    Animal/veterinary work experience

    Animal and veterinary experience is considered to evaluate the applicant's personal qualities and motivation to be a veterinarian.

    Animal experience includes caring for and handling animals in a kennel or animal shelter. It also includes any other experience that was not under the direct supervision of a veterinarian, such as FFA and 4-H projects. Veterinary experience is hours spent working under the direct supervisions of a veterinarian, whether in a clinical or research environment, paid or volunteer. **Applicants must have more than 50 hours worth of veterinary experience in order to qualify for an interview.**

    Points are assigned based on the number of hours worked and the variety of environments in which the hours were obtained. These two experiences are scored separately, so applicants should obtain experience in both areas. For example, an applicant who worked for a veterinarian should include time spent cleaning stalls or cages as animal experience and time spent with the veterinarian as veterinary experience.

Summary of Admission Procedure

Timetable
    Application deadline: October 1
    Date interviews are held: December–mid-February
    Date acceptances mailed: mid-March
    School begins: late August

Deposit (to hold place in class): none required.

Deferments: requests for deferments will be considered on a case-by-case basis.

Evaluation criteria
    Academic performance
    Test scores
    Interview
    Personal statement
    Evaluations (3 evaluations are required. No letters of support/
        recommendation are needed)

Semester course load and postacademic challenge
Leadership and experience

2009–2010 admissions summary

	Number of Applicants	Number of New Entrants
Resident	351	122
Nonresident	90	10
Total:	441	132

Expenses for the 2008–2009 Academic Year

Tuition and fees

Resident	$14,374.00
Nonresident	$25,174.00

Tufts University

Office of Admissions
Cummings School of Veterinary Medicine
200 Westboro Road
Tufts University
North Grafton MA 01536
Telephone: (508) 839-7920
Email: vetadmissions@tufts.edu
www.tufts.edu/vet/

Tufts University is located near Boston, where athletic and cultural activities abound. The Cummings School of Veterinary Medicine provides an exciting biomedical environment for the study of modern veterinary medicine. Signature programs include wildlife medicine, international veterinary medicine, and equine sports medicine. Issues related to the ethical dimensions of veterinary medicine, including animal welfare, are an integral aspect of the curriculum. Hands-on learning begins in the first year and continues throughout the next three years. Many opportunities exist outside of formal courses for hands-on work in hospitals and research laboratories. The Hospital for Large Animals, Foster Hospital for Small Animals, the Ambulatory Service, and the Wildlife Clinic provide a rich mixture of horses, cats, dogs, cattle, sheep, goats, and native wildlife. Our large caseload, typically ranked among the top three schools in the country, provides exciting learning opportunities for students.

Application Information

For specific application information (availability, deadlines, fees, and VMCAS participation), please refer to the contact information listed above.

Residency implications: Massachusetts residents make up about half of each class. All others considered for the remaining spaces. Tufts contracts with Maine (1), New Hampshire (1–2), and New Jersey (4).

Prerequisites for Admission

Course requirements and semesters
Biology (with laboratory)	2
Inorganic chemistry (with laboratory)	2
Organic chemistry (with laboratory)	2
Physics	2
Mathematics	2
Genetics, unless included in biology	1

Biochemistry	1
English composition	2
Social and behavioral sciences	2
Humanities and fine arts	2

Required undergraduate GPA: no minimum GPA required. The average GPA for the class admitted in 2009 was 3.66.

AP credit policy: must appear on official college transcripts and be equivalent to the appropriate college-level coursework.

Course completion deadline: prerequisite courses must be completed by the time of matriculation into the DVM program.

Standardized examinations: Graduate Record Examinations (GRE®), general test, is required. The most recent acceptable test date for applicants to the class of 2015 is November 2010. The oldest acceptable scores must be within 5 years of the application deadline. Average GRE scores for the class of 2013 were verbal 610, quantitative 710, and analytical 4.5.

Additional requirements and considerations
    Animal/veterinary/biomedical research experience
    Letters of Evaluation (3 required)
        advisor/faculty members
        veterinarian/research scientist
    Essays
    Interview
    Extracurricular /community service activities
    Leadership potential

Summary of Admission Procedure

Timetable
    Application deadline: November 1
    Date interviews are held: December, February
    Date acceptances mailed: March
    School begins: late August

Deposit (to hold place in class): $500.00.

Deferments: requests for deferment are handled on a case-by-case basis.

Evaluation criteria
Tufts' admission procedure consists of a review of the application and an interview of selected applicants.

2009–2010 admissions summary

	Number of Applicants	Number of New Entrants
Total:	704	87

Expenses for the 2009–2010 Academic Year

Tuition and fees

Resident	$36,468.00
Contract*	varies
Nonresident	$39,426.00

* For further information, see the listing of contracting states and provinces.

Dual-Degree Program

Combined DVM–graduate degree programs are available.

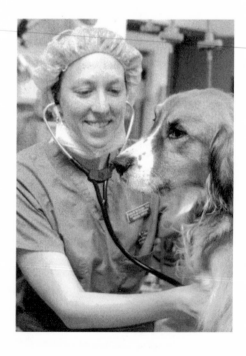

Veterinary medical students find their clinical rounds not only educational but also personally satisfying. Photo courtesy of Tufts University Cummings School of Veterinary Medicine.

Tuskegee University

Office of Veterinary Admissions and Recruitment
Tuskegee University School of Veterinary Medicine
Tuskegee AL 36088
Telephone: (334) 727-8460

Tuskegee University School of Veterinary Medicine is located in Tuskegee, Alabama, a city of about 13,000. The city is located about 40 miles east of Montgomery and 40 miles west of Columbus, Georgia. Summers are hot with moderate to mild humidity, and winters are moderate. Recreational facilities, lakes, parks and other educational institutions are located nearby.

The university was founded by Booker T. Washington in 1881, and a large part of the campus has been declared a historical site by the United States Department of the Interior. The veterinary school was established in 1945 and over 70% of African-American veterinarians in the United States receive their professional training at Tuskegee University.

Application Information

For specific application information (availability, deadlines, fees, and VM-CAS), please refer to the contact information listed above, or visit the online application process at: www.onemedicine.tuskegee.edu.

Residency implications: applications are accepted with special consideration given to Alabama residents and those who have residency in the following contract states, Kentucky, New Jersey, South Carolina, and West Virginia.

Prerequisites for Admission

Course requirements and semester hours

English composition/communications	6
Mathematics (algebra and trigonometry)	6
Chemistry (minimum)	
Organic chemistry (with laboratory)	8
Biochemistry (laboratory recommended but not required)	4
Physics* (with laboratories)	8
Biological science (above 300 level)	
Advanced biology**	9
Free electives	8
(advanced biological science—optional)	
Animal science	9
(includes poultry and animal nutrition)	

| Social science and humanities | 6 |
| Electives—liberal arts | 6 |

* One academic year

** Advanced biology courses, e.g., ecology, physiology, immunology, zoology, microbiology, genetics, anatomy, physiology, and histology

Required undergraduate GPA: the cumulative and science GPA requirement is 2.7 on a 4.00 scale.

Course completion deadline: prerequisite courses must be completed by end of May.

Standardized examinations: Graduate Record Examination (GRE®) or Medical College Admission Test (MCAT), any of which must be taken within 3 years of application, is required. Must be completed by Oct. 1.

Summary of Admission Procedure

Timetable
    Application deadline: October 1
    Date interviews are held: January–February
    Date acceptances mailed: April 15
    School begins: late August

Deferments: one-year deferments are considered on a case-by-case basis.

Evaluation criteria
The following items are taken into consideration: academic record, academic trends, letters of recommendation, work experience, and test scores.

	% weight
Grades	60
Test scores	2
Animal/veterinary experience	1
Interview	15
References - 2 science professors, 1 veterinarian	1
Essay - 1 page handwritten, see application	1

Number of available seats - 65

Expenses for the 2008–2009 Academic Year

Tuition and fees

In state	$9,425.00
Out of state	$13,800.00
Technology fee	$150.00
I.D. fee	$30.00

If admitted, additional fees and expenses are required.

Dual-Degree Programs

Combined DVM–graduate degree programs are available.

Virginia-Maryland Regional College of Veterinary Medicine

Admissions Coordinator
Virginia-Maryland Regional College of Veterinary Medicine
Blacksburg VA 24061
Telephone: (540) 231-4699
Fax: (540) 231-9290
Email: dvmadmit@vt.edu
www.vetmed.vt.edu

The Virginia-Maryland Regional College of Veterinary Medicine is situated on 3 distinct campuses. The main campus is at Virginia Tech in Blacksburg, Virginia, a community with a population of about 40,000 situated on a high plateau in southwestern Virginia between the Blue Ridge and Allegheny Mountains. Its residents enjoy a wide range of educational, social, recreational, and cultural opportunities. In addition to the Blacksburg campus, the Equine Medical Center campus is in Leesburg, Virginia, and the University of Maryland is at College Park. The college received full accreditation in 1993 from the American Veterinary Medical Association.

In recognition of a need for veterinarians trained in both basic and clinical sciences, the college offers students the opportunity to participate in graduate studies and receive appropriate advanced training to conduct research in basic or clinical disciplines. Nearly 25 percent of the nation's veterinarians work in areas other than private practice, such as government and corporate veterinary medicine. Through the assistance of a grant from the Pew Charitable Trusts, the college has established the Center for Public and Corporate Veterinary Medicine, which is a national resource for training veterinarians for the wide variety of careers in this area of the profession.

Application Information

For specific application information (availability, deadlines, fees, and VMCAS participation), please refer to the contact information listed above.

Residency implications: 50 positions are reserved for Virginia residents, and 30 positions for Maryland residents. Up to 15 additional positions may be filled by nonresidents.

Prerequisites for Admission

Course requirements and semester hours

Biological sciences (with laboratories)	8
Organic chemistry (with laboratories)	8
Physics (with laboratories)	8
Biochemistry	3
English (composition, 3 credit hours)	6
Humanities/social science	6
Mathematics (algebra, geometry, trigonometry, calculus)	6

Students must earn a C– or better in all required courses.

Science courses taken 7 or more years ago may be repeated or substituted with higher-level courses with the written consent of the admissions committee.

Required undergraduate GPA: to be considered for admission, applicants must have a cumulative GPA of at least 2.80 on a 4.00 scale upon completion of a minimum of 2 academic years of full-time study (60 semester/90 quarter hours) at an accredited college or university. Alternatively, a 3.30 GPA in the last 2 years (60 semester hours) will qualify a student who does not have a 2.80 GPA overall. All courses taken during this 2-year period must be junior or senior level. The mean GPA of those accepted into the class of 2012 was 3.5.

Advanced placement credit for 1 semester of English will be accepted if the additional required hours are composition or technical writing and are taken at a college or university.

Advanced placement credit or credit by examination for preveterinary course requirements will be accepted. Those credits must appear on the applicant's college transcript. Advanced placement credits will not be calculated in grade point averages and no grade assigned. No course substitutions will be allowed for AP credit or credit by examination.

Course completion deadline: required courses must be completed by the end of the spring term of the year in which matriculation occurs.

Standardized examinations: Graduate Record Examination (GRE®) is required. The GRE must have been taken within the last 5 years.

Additional requirements and considerations

Maturity and a broad cultural perspective

Motivation and dedication to a career in veterinary medicine

Evidence of potential, and appreciation of the career opportunities for veterinarians, as indicated by:

1. Clinical veterinary experience (private practice)
2. Animal experience in addition to time spent working with a veterinarian
3. Biomedical/research experience (such as working with veterinarians or other biomedically trained individuals in health care, government, research laboratories, industrial, or corporate settings.)
4. Extramural activities, achievements, honors
5. Communication skills
6. References

Summary of Admission Procedure

Timetable
> VMCAS application deadline: Friday, October 1, 2010 12:00 PM (noon) Eastern Time
> Supplemental application deadline: October 1
> Date interviews are held: February
> Date acceptances mailed: early March
> School begins: mid-August

Deposit (to hold place in class): $450.00 for Maryland and Virginia residents; $1,000.00 for nonresidents.

Deferments: case-by-case basis if a candidate has extenuating circumstances beyond his or her control.

Evaluation criteria
The admission procedure is comprised of an initial screening of applicants, an interview of selected applicants, and a final review of the dossiers of all interviewees.

	% weight
Academics	50
Cumulative GPA, required science GPA, last 45 semester-hour GPA, GRE® aptitude	
Background	25
Related animal experience; veterinary experience; research, industrial, and commercial experience; activities, achievements, and awards; narrative and personal references	
Interviews	25

	Number of Applicants	Number of New Entrants
Resident		
Maryland	120	30
Virginia	185	50
Nonresident	<u>589</u>	<u>15</u>
Total:	894	95

Expenses for the 2009–2010 Academic Year

Tuition and fees
Resident	$18,415.00
Nonresident	$40,607.00

Dual-Degree Programs

Combined DVM–graduate degree programs are available.

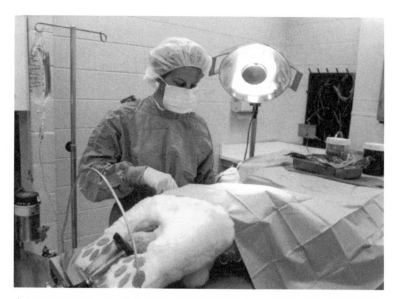

A junior veterinary student practices suturing techniques during the "Teddy Bear Repair Clinic" at the Virginia-Maryland Regional College of Veterinary Medicine's annual Open House. Photo courtesy of Biomedical Media Center, VMRCVM.

Washington State University

Office of Student Services
College of Veterinary Medicine
Washington State University
P. O. Box 647012
Pullman WA 99164-7012
Telephone: (509) 335-1532
Email: admissions@vetmed.wsu.edu
Website: www.vetmed.wsu.edu

Washington State University is located in Pullman, a city of 27,000 people situated in southeastern Washington. WSU is a member of the PAC-10 athletic conference. The area has much to offer those who seek a lifestyle that combines a beautiful country setting with the benefits of two major universities (University of Idaho is 9 miles away). With a true four season climate and beautiful rivers and nearby mountains, there are excellent recreational activities available ranging from hiking, mountain biking, skiing and snowboarding, to fishing, camping and whitewater rafting.

The College of Veterinary Medicine was founded in 1899 and is one of the oldest colleges of veterinary medicine in the country. Five major buildings house the departments of veterinary clinical sciences, comparative anatomy pharmacology and physiology, and microbiology and pathology, along with the Washington Animal Disease Diagnostic Laboratory. The faculty and staff of the Veterinary Teaching Hospital are considered leaders in the field of veterinary diagnostic imaging. The well regarded oncology unit offers an active clinical service delivering medical and radiation oncology to a wide variety of companion animals. The hospital attracts a large and diverse caseload for the DVM educational program. The veterinary teaching program also allows for students to take advantage of numerous off-campus clinical opportunities in all areas of veterinary medicine.

The college is a leader in the development of programs to promote and enhance emotional intelligence, leadership and communication skills. The School for Global Animal Health, the first of its kind in North America, is serving as the centerpiece of the college's expanded research on animal diseases that directly impact human health. M.S. and Ph.D. degrees are offered by each of the three academic departments in the College of Veterinary Medicine. For those DVM students interested in gaining research experience, numerous opportunities exist, including the competitive Research Scholars Program, which is designed to encourage the exploration of research careers in veterinary medicine. A combined DVM-extended MPH degree program is available through a cooperative program with University of Washington.

Application Information

For the most current application information (availability, deadlines, fees, and VMCAS participation), please refer to the contact information listed above.

Residency implications: In general, first preference is given to qualified applicants who are residents of Washington or Idaho, as well as qualified applicants certified by WICHE contract states. Second preference is given to qualified applicants from non-service area states and non-certified applicants from WICHE states.

Prerequisites for Admission

Course requirements and semester hours

Biology (with lab)	8
Inorganic Chemistry (with lab)	8
Organic Chemistry (with lab)	4
Physics (with lab)	4
Math (precalculus or higher)	3
Genetics	4
Biochemistry	3
Statistical Methods	3
Arts/Humanities/Social Sciences/History*	21
English Composition/Communication*	6
Total	64

These requirements will be waived if a student has a bachelor's degree.

Required undergraduate GPA: none; a minimum overall GPA of 3.20 on a 4.00 scale is recommended.

AP credit policy: Must meet Washington State University requirements.

Course completion deadline: Prerequisite courses must be completed by June 15 prior to entry.

Standardized examinations: Graduate Record Examination (GRE®), general test, is required. Test scores older than 5 years will not be accepted.

Additional requirements and considerations
>   Animal/veterinary/research/work experience
>   Recommendations (3 required, one by a veterinarian)
>   Extracurricular and/or community service activities

Summary of Admission Procedure

Timetable
>   VMCAS application deadline: Friday, October 1, 2010 12:00 PM (noon)
>   Eastern Time; WSU Supplemental - October 8, 2010 by 5pm PST
>   Date interviews are held: January–February

Date acceptances mailed: January–April
School begins: late August

Deposit (to hold place in class): None required.

Deferments: Considered on a case-by-case basis.

Evaluation criteria
Applicants will be selected based upon ability to successfully complete the program and demonstration of the qualities of a good veterinarian. Academic criteria include grades, quality and rigor of academic program and GRE test scores. Nonacademic factors include animal/veterinary/research/work experience, honors & awards, community service, extracurricular activities, essay, letters of recommendation; other factors include maturity, integrity, compassion, communication skills, and desire to contribute to society. An interview will be required for Washington and Idaho residents, as well as for out-of-area applicants. WICHE applicants are ranked for WICHE funding using the same criteria above minus the interview.

2008–2009 admissions summary

	Number of Applicants	Number of New Entrants
Washington	143	56
Idaho	42	11
WICHE†	204	16
Nonresident	463	15
Total:	852	98

† For further information, see the listing of contracting states and provinces.

Expenses for the 2009–2010 Academic Year

Tuition and fees

Resident (WA, ID, and WICHE supported)	$18,332.00
Nonresident	$45,342.00

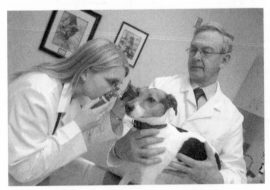

During their 4th year in the DVM program at Washington State University, students hone their physical exam and other clinical skills. Photo courtesy of: Washington State University College of Veterinary Medicine

Western University of Health Sciences

Office of Admission
College of Veterinary Medicine
Western University of Health Sciences
309 East 2nd Street
Pomona, CA 91766-1854
Phone: (909) 623-6116 FAX: (909) 469-5570
E-mail: admissions@westernu.edu
Web site: http://www.prospective.westernu.edu/veterinary/requirements

Western University of Health Sciences is an independent, accredited, non-profit university incorporated in the State of California, dedicated to educating compassionate and scientifically competent health professionals who value diversity and a humanistic approach to patient care. The university, located in the San Gabriel Valley of Southern California, about 30 miles east of Los Angeles, grants post baccalaureate professional degrees in nine colleges: the College of Podiatric Medicine, the College of Dental Medicine, the College of Optometry, the Graduate College of Biomedical Sciences, the College of Allied Health Professions, the College of Graduate Nursing, the College of Osteopathic Medicine of the Pacific, the College of Pharmacy, and the College of Veterinary Medicine. The AVMA Council on Education granted the College of Veterinary Medicine limited accreditation status in 2008. Western U's CVM admitted its charter class Fall 2003. The founding principles of the College of Veterinary Medicine include:

1) *Commitment to student-centered, life-long learning.*
   The curriculum is designed to teach students to find and critically evaluate information, to enhance student cooperative learning, and to provide an environment for professional development.

2) *Commitment to a Reverence for Life philosophy in teaching veterinary medicine.*
   The College strives to make the educational experience one that enhances moral development of its students and is respectful to all animals and people involved in its programs.

3) *Commitment to excellence of student education through strategic partnerships in the public and private veterinary sectors.*
   This commitment seeks to maximize the learning experience in veterinary clinical practice and to educate practice-ready veterinarians capable of functioning independently upon graduation.

Phase I (Years 1 & 2): Basic and clinical veterinary science education using problem-based learning modules, a veterinary issues seminar series, a molecular biology seminar series, and an experiential clinical skills course.

123

Phase II (Year 3): Required rotations in thirteen different areas of veterinary medicine in regional veterinary practices or institutions including some rotations conducted on campus.

Phase III (Year 4): Selective rotations in regional, national or international specialty practices, veterinary teaching hospitals, or public/private institutions to be determined by students' career goals.

Application Information

For specific application information (availability, deadlines, fees, and VMCAS participation), please refer to the contact information listed previously.

Residency implications: applicants from all states as well as international applicants will be considered. In-state and out-of-state applicants are given equal consideration.

Prerequisites for Admissions

Course requirements[1]:

	Semester Units	Quarter Units
Organic chemistry (including laboratory)	3	4
Biochemistry or Physiological Chemistry[2,3]	3	4
Biological & Life Sciences[3,4,5]	9	12
(must be upper-division Biological & Life Sciences and include one upper-division laboratory course)*		
Microbiology[3,5]	3	4
Physiology[3,5]	3	4
Genetics or Molecular Biology[3,5]	3	4
General physics (including laboratory)	6	8
Statistics or Calculus[2]	3	4
English composition	6	8
Public Speaking or Small Group Communication	3	4
Psychology or sociology	3	4
Humanities/social sciences	9	12

* Ex: biology, physiology, anatomy, cell biology, embryology, zoology

1,2,3,4,5: See Course completion deadline on following page for details.

Required undergraduate GPA: Applicants must have a minimum overall, prerequisite science and prerequisite GPA of 2.75 (undergraduate and graduate) at the time of application to be considered for admission. Prerequisite courses must be completed with a grade of C (or its equivalent) or higher.

AP credit policy: must appear on official college transcripts and be equivalent to the appropriate college-level coursework. AP test subject and number of credits must also be specified on the transcript.

Course completion deadline: (1) All courses must be completed at a regionally accredited college or university in the United States. Exceptions will be made on a case-by-case basis. Coursework completed outside the U.S. (including Canada) must be evaluated by a WesternU approved evaluation service. All required courses must be completed by the end of the spring term of planned matriculation year. Failure to satisfactorily complete prerequisites with a grade of C or better will result in the loss of a candidate's seat in the class. One course cannot be used to satisfy more than one prerequisite. (2) Must be a course designed or specified for science majors. (3) These required courses must have been completed no more than 8 years prior to the date of matriculation at WesternU-CVM. Classes taken after August 1, 2003, will be considered within the 8-year time limit and may be applied toward the prerequisites for the class entering Fall 2011. (4) While not specifically required, courses in anatomy, nutrition and embryology are strongly encouraged. (5) All except two of these courses must be completed by the end of the fall term immediately prior to the planned year of matriculation at WesternU-CVM.

Standardized examinations: Graduate Record Examination (GRE®), general test, or Medical College Admissions Test (MCAT) is required. Test scores must be postmarked by the October 15, 2010, supplemental application deadline. Test scores older than five years prior to the planned year of matriculation are not acceptable.

Additional requirements and considerations:
> Animal experience: must total at least 500 hours of hands-on experience that goes beyond observation. Appropriate venues include but are not limited to: animal medical environment/ veterinary practice; commercial animal production; regulatory animal control; animal entertainment or research environment.
> Recommendations/evaluations: 3 are required from among the following: previous employers, supervisors of extended volunteer activities, academic personnel.
> Interview

Summary of Admissions Procedure

Timetable
> VMCAS application deadline: Friday, October 1, 2010 12:00 PM (noon) Eastern Time

Supplemental application deadline: postmarked on or before October
15
Date interviews are held: January–February
Date acceptances mailed: March
School begins: August

Deposit (to hold place in class): $500.

Deferments: request for deferments will be considered on a case-by-case basis.

Evaluation criteria:
Academic achievement
Standardized test performance
Animal experience
Letters of reference
Interview
Other supporting material

2009–2010 admissions summary

	Number of Applicants	Number of New Entrants
Resident	305	70
Nonresident	433	30
Total:	738	100

Expenses for the 2009–2010 Academic Year

Tuition and fees
Resident	$40,105.00
Nonresident	$40,105.00

University of Wisconsin

Office of Academic Affairs
School of Veterinary Medicine
2015 Linden Drive
University of Wisconsin-Madison
Madison WI 53706-1102
Telephone: (608) 263-2525
www.vetmed.wisc.edu/oaa

The University of Wisconsin is located in Madison, the state capital, which has a population of about 208,000. Consistently ranked among the nation's "most livable" cities, its hilly terrain, scattered parks, and woodlands saturate the urban setting with a friendly neighborhood atmosphere. Centered on a narrow isthmus among 4 scenic lakes, the city is a recreational paradise. The university sprawls over 900 acres along Lake Mendota and its student population is nearly 45,000. It has rated among the top 10 universities academically since 1910 and is third in the country in volume of research activity.

The School of Veterinary Medicine facility has a modern veterinary teaching hospital, modern equipment, and high-quality lab space for teaching and research. The curriculum provides a broad education in veterinary medicine with learning experiences in food animal medicine and other specialty areas. The school pioneered a unique senior rotation in ambulatory service for fourth-year students where they experience the life and work of a veterinarian specializing in large-animal medicine by working in one of 22 practices near Madison. The school has an outstanding research program and many faculty members have joint appointments with the College of Agriculture, the School of Medicine and Public Health, the Regional Primate Center, the McArdle Cancer Research Institute, the National Wildlife Health Laboratory, and the North Central Dairy Forage Center. These outside links provide research and job opportunities for students.

Application Information

For specific application information (availability, deadlines, fees, and VMCAS participation), please refer to the contact information listed above.

Residency implications: between 60 and 70 Wisconsin residents will be accepted. Wisconsin has no contractual agreements, but may accept 10–20 nonresidents. Applicants who can claim legal residency or domicile in more than one state should contact the school.

Prerequisites for Admission

Applicants must complete a minimum of 60 semester credits of college coursework. The 60 credits include the required 40–43 credits of coursework listed below, plus a minimum of 17 credits of elective coursework left to the student's discretion. The 17 elective credits allow the student to meet personal and academic goals and objectives while preparing for admission to veterinary school.

Course requirements and semester hours

General biology or zoology, introductory animal biology course (with laboratory)	5
General and qualitative chemistry, 2-semester lecture series (with laboratory)	8
Organic chemistry, 1-semester lecture satisfying bio-chemistry prerequisite	3
Biochemistry (organic chemistry must be prerequisite)	3
English composition or journalism	6

Must include completion of:
- satisfactory score on a college English placement exam, or
- an introductory English composition course,

plus completion of one of the following:
- an English composition or journalism course graded on the basis of writing skills, or
- evidence that writing skills were included in the grading of a specific college-level course

Genetics or animal breeding, must include principles of heredity and preferably molecular mechanisms	3
General physics, 2-semester lecture series	6
Statistics, introductory course	3
Social sciences/humanities, any elective courses in social science or the humanities	6

Required undergraduate GPA: A minimum grade of C (2.0) must be earned in all required courses, including courses completed after application. The mean cumulative GPA for the class of 2013 was 3.57 for residents and 3.73 for non-residents.

AP credit policy: must appear on official college transcripts and be equivalent to the appropriate college-level coursework.

Course completion deadline: all coursework must be completed no later than the spring 2011 term prior to admission to the fall 2011 term. For fall 2011 admissions cycle, applicants can have no more than four outstanding required courses at the time of application, with no more than two of those four to be completed during the spring semester. Applicants are encouraged to prepare themselves for the DVM curriculum by taking additional upper-level science courses such as anatomy, physiology, microbiology, or cell/molecular biology.

Standardized examinations: Graduate Record Examination (GRE®), general test, is required. All applicants are required to take or retake the GRE, including the writing assessment. The GRE may be taken no later than October 1, 2010. The mean score for the class of 2013 for the verbal and quantitative portions combined was 1227 for residents and 1249 for nonresidents.

A test of English as a foreign language (TOEFL, MELAB or IELTS scores may be submitted) is required for applicants for whom English is a second language and have not completed an undergraduate education at an English-speaking college or university. The minimum scores accepted are as follows: internet TOEFL=100, computer TOEFL=250, paper TOEFL=600, MELAB=84, IELTS=7. This must be taken no later than **October 1, 2010.** Please see Web site for additional information.

Additional requirements and considerations
    Veterinary medical experience
    Animal contact and work experience
    Other preparatory experience
    College degrees earned
    Extracurricular activities
    Recommendations/evaluations (3 required)
    Honors/awards
    Diversity of background and experiences
    Personal statement

Summary of Admission Procedure

Timetable
    VMCAS application deadline: Friday, October 1, 2010 12:00 PM
        (noon) Eastern Time
    Interviews: none
    Date acceptances mailed: mid-March
    School begins: late August/early September

Deposit (to hold place in class): none required.

Deferments: are considered on an individual basis by the Admissions Committee and may be granted for extenuating circumstances.

Evaluation criteria
There is a 2-part admission procedure. For the fall 2009 application year, the class was selected based upon the following comparative evaluation:

129

1. *Evaluation of academic record*
   Undergraduate cumulative GPA
   Required course GPA
   Most recent 30 semester credit GPA
   GRE® test scores
2. *Evaluation of personal experience and characteristics*
   Animal and veterinary work experience
   Other preparatory experience (includes extracurricular activities)
   Personal history/academic performance (summary category to include
      review of academic history, academic achievements, diversity of
      background, etc.)
   Reference letters

2008–2009 admissions summary

	Number of Applicants	Number of New Entrants
Resident	188	60
Nonresident	942	20
Total:	1,130	80

Expenses for the 2009–2010 Academic Year

Tuition and fees
| Resident | $17,715.00 |
| Nonresident | $25,787.00 |

Dual-Degree Programs

Combined DVM–graduate degree programs are available.

INTERNATIONAL VETERINARY MEDICAL SCHOOLS

University College Dublin
Veterinary Medicine Degree Programme

VMCAS Veterinary Medicine Applications
UCD Admissions Office
Tierney Building
University College Dublin
Belfield, Dublin 4
Ireland
Tel: 00 353 1 716 1555
Email: onlineapps@ucd.ie
http://www.ucd.ie/vetmed/

University College Dublin (UCD) traces its origins to the Catholic University of Ireland founded in 1854 by Cardinal John Henry Newman, author of the celebrated "The Idea of a University." Since then, the University has played a central role in Ireland's advancement as a dynamic and highly successful European state and has established a long and distinguished tradition of service to scholarship and the community.

UCD is the sole provider of a veterinary medicine degree programme on the island of Ireland, and enjoys a long and proud tradition in the provision of veterinary education. Students of the veterinary medicine programme benefit from the outstanding facilities of the purpose-designed UCD Veterinary Sciences Centre and UCD Veterinary Hospital on the main university campus at Belfield, Dublin (commissioned in 2002). Located on a 132 Ha site 5km south of Dublin's City Centre, UCD is Ireland's largest university with over 23,000 students. The veterinary facilities are state-of-the-art. As part of the UCD College of Life Sciences we provide the ideal environment for students and staff to work together to push back the frontiers of knowledge in veterinary research, thus advancing animal health, animal welfare, and human health.

Programme/Syllabus

Our programme is designed to educate you to the best international standards in veterinary medicine and to prepare you for entry to any branch of the veterinary profession. Veterinary medicine is concerned with the promotion of the health and welfare of animals of special importance to society. This involves the care of healthy and sick animals, the prevention, recognition, control and treatment of their diseases and the welfare and productivity of livestock. Veterinarians also safeguard human health through prevention and control of diseases transmitted from animals to man, through ensuring the safety of foods of animal origin, and through advancing the science and art of comparative medicine.

Veterinary graduates may work in private practice (companion animals, food animals, horses, exotics, pr a mixture of these), in government service (animal health, food safety, public health), in research or in industry. Our veterinary programme is accredited by the Veterinary Council of Ireland, the American Veterinary Medical Association, and the European Association of Establishments in Veterinary Education.

A new 4-year programme specifically for graduate entrants commenced in September 2009. US applicants through VMCAS are eligible to apply to enter this programme provided they have the prerequisites as outlined below. Further curricular details are published on our web site, www.ucd.ie/vetmed.

The Programme is organised into two stages- Stage 1 comprising the first two semesters and Stage 2 the remaining 6 semesters. In Semesters 1 and 2 of the programme students will build on their knowledge of the basic biological sciences by taking modules designed to demonstrate how this knowledge is applied in the practice of veterinary medicine, and gain a firm grounding in animal welfare, behaviour and handling. A key objective will be to ensure that students have the required knowledge, skills and competences to progress to Stage 2. As the programme progresses students will learn clinical skills and study each of the clinical sciences using a "body systems" approach. The final year of the programme consists of clinical rotations in UCD's veterinary hospital where students have the opportunity to work alongside experienced and specialist staff clinicians, and participate in patient care and client communication. Each student has a personalized timetable ensuring that they participate in rotations in Large and Small Animal Surgeries, Diagnostic Imaging, Anesthesiology, Small and Large Animal Medicine, Emergency Medicine, Clinical Reproduction, Herd Health, Population Medicine, Diagnostic Pathology and Clinical Pathology. Assessments at the end of this clinical year are through Objective Structured Clinical Examinations (OSCEs) and Clinical Proficiency Examinations (CPEs). Throughout the programme students are required to participate in extra-mural studies. In the early years, this consists of gaining experience in the handling and management of farm and companion animals, and in later years, of working with veterinarians in practice (clinical extra-mural experience). Some of this experience can be undertaken in the US or elsewhere, according to student preference.

Application Information

For specific application information (availability, fees and VMCAS participation), please refer to the contact information listed above. For further information on entry to the Republic of Ireland, please refer to www.educationireland.ie. Students must also be able to ensure adequate financial support for the duration of their programme.

Prerequisites for Admission

Course requirements

4-Year Graduate Entry Programme

Candidates who have studied and will complete a degree in an appropriate biological science may be considered for the 4- year Graduate programme in Veterinary Medicine with the award of MVB.

Required undergraduate GPA: 3.2 (on 4.0-point scale)

Course completion deadline: all required courses should be completed prior to August of the year of admission.

5-Year Undergraduate Programme MVB: Those candidates with a nonscience degree would be considered for first year entry to the 5-year MVB programme, provided they have gained high grades in the science subjects, including chemistry and biology.

Standardized examinations: none required. However, if the applicant already has a GRE® score, then he/she is asked but not required to send it in.

Additional requirements and considerations
Applicants are also expected to have gained relevant work experience of handling animals. This should, where possible, include not only seeing veterinary practice, but also spending time on livestock farms and other animal establishments.

Summary of Admission Procedure

Timetable
> VMCAS application deadline: Friday, October 1, 2010 12:00 PM
> (noon) Eastern Time
> Date offers mailed: Late January/Early February
> Term begins: early September

Deposit (to hold place in class): €2,000 euros, required by early March

Deferments: Not applicable

Evaluation criteria
  Academic performance
  References/evaluations (minimum 2 required-one from academic
    science source and one from a veterinary surgeon)
  1 page personal statement
  Animal & Veterinary Experience

2008–2009 admissions summary (for entry in 2009)

	Number of Applicants	Number of New Entrants
In-province	791	92
International	135	32
Total	926	124

Expenses for the 2010–2011*

Annual tuition and fees
  EU Graduate   19,500 euros
  Non EU Graduate   33,500 euros

* For up-to-date information on fees and all further information regarding admission to the University College Dublin, please visit our web site www.ucd.ie.

University of Edinburgh
Royal (Dick) School of Veterinary Studies

BVM&S Admissions Office
Royal (Dick) School of Veterinary Studies
The University of Edinburgh
Easter Bush Veterinary Centre
Roslin EH25 9RG
Scotland, UK
Tel: +44 (0)131 651 7305
Fax: +44 (0)131 650 6585
Email: geraldine.giannopoulos@ed.ac.uk
http://www.ed.ac.uk/schools-departments/vet

The Royal (Dick) School of Veterinary Studies, established in 1823, was the first veterinary school in Scotland, and the second to be established in the UK. The long-standing involvement of Edinburgh with veterinary education, where tradition is mixed with cutting-edge veterinary teaching, benefits from a closely-knit collegial community of "Dick" vet students. As one of only 14 international vet schools with AVMA accreditation, the veterinary degree course at Edinburgh (BVM&S) provides an excellent foundation for a subsequent career in veterinary practice or one of the many related career opportunities, such as biomedical research. The academic and research environment in Edinburgh is internationally recognised for encouraging excellence in a broad base of teaching and learning. The school is on 2 sites: one in central Edinburgh and the other at the Easter Bush Veterinary Centre in nearby Roslin, approximately 7 miles south of the city. In 2011, the new Veterinary School Teaching Building is scheduled for completion, meaning the whole School will be located at Easter Bush.

The city of Edinburgh, the capital of Scotland, is one of Europe's most handsome cities. The beauty of its setting and its architecture, allied with its intellectual traditions, have earned the title of "Athens of the North" for what is still a compact city of some 500,000 people. It is a city of noted buildings, fine gardens, and open spaces, including Holyrood Park—one of the largest city centre natural parks in Europe—and Princes Street Gardens, between the Old and New Towns. The city offers students a rich mix of academic, social and allied facilities—libraries, museums and art galleries, concert halls, theatres and cinemas. The city has easy access to coastline, lochs, mountains and countryside, with ready-made opportunities for open-air sports and recreation.

Further details on the BVM&S degree programme, the School and its facilities can be found by visiting http://www.ed.ac.uk/schools-departments/vet

Application Information

For specific application information (availability, deadlines, fees and VMCAS participation), please refer to the contact information listed above.

Residency implications: For full details and further information on entry to the UK, please refer to http://www.ukvisas.gov.uk. Please note that students must be able to ensure adequate financial support for the duration of their course.

Prerequisites for Admission

Course requirements

5-Year BVM&S Programme:

Applicants are expected to have completed a minimum of at least 2 years of a preveterinary or science course at college or university. A minimum of one year (2 semesters or 3 terms) in chemistry, and additional courses in biology, physics and/or mathematics are required. All applicants are required to have gained high grades in the science subjects, especially chemistry. U.S. applicants should have an overall minimum grade point average of 3.4 (4-point scale), with greater than 3.0 in science courses which have been completed.

Those candidates with a nonscience degree would be considered for first-year entry to the 5-year BVM&S course, provided they have gained high grades in the science subjects, including chemistry and biology.

4-Year Graduate Entry Programme:

Candidates who have studied and will complete a degree in an appropriate biological science may be considered for the 4-year BVM&S programme (Graduate Entry Programme).

Required undergraduate GPA: 3.4 (on 4.0-point scale)

Course completion deadline: all required courses should be completed prior to August of the year of admission.

Standardized examinations: none required. However, if the applicant already has a GRE® score, then he/she is asked but not required to send it in.

Additional requirements and considerations
Applicants are also expected to have gained relevant work experience of handling animals. This should, where possible, include not only seeing veterinary practice, but also spending time on livestock farms and other animal establishments.

Summary of Admission Procedure

Timetable

    VMCAS application deadline: Friday, October 1, 2010 12:00 PM
       (noon) Eastern Time

    Receptions: early–mid-February (held in the U.S.)

    Date acceptances mailed: early April at the latest

    School begins: mid-September or early August (for GEP entrants)

Deposit (to hold place in class): £1,500, required by early May

Deferments: Not applicable

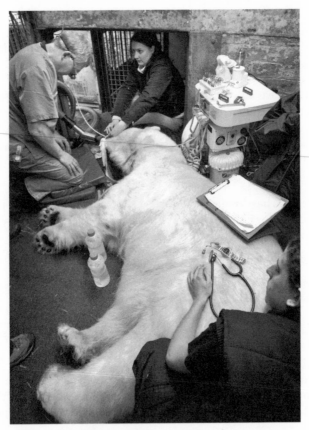

Zoo Veterinary Medicine is just one of the University of
Edinburgh's many strengths. Photo by Paul Dodds, courtesy of
University of Edinburgh.

Evaluation criteria
　　Academic performance
　　Animal/veterinary experience
　　Personal statement
　　Motivation
　　References/Evaluations (minimum 2 required—one from academic
　　　science source and one from a veterinary surgeon)

2008–2009 admissions summary (for entry in 2009)*

	Number of Applicants	*Number of New Entrants*
In-province	881	126
International	307	45
Total	1,188	171

Expenses for the 2010–2011 Academic Year*

Tuition and fees

Resident	residents of the UK are government-funded
International	£22,200
	(fixed for duration of course)

* For up-to-date information on fees and all further information regarding admission to the School, please visit our website www.ed.ac.uk/schools-departments/vet

University of Glasgow

Mrs. Joyce Wason
Director of Admissions & Student Services Manager
University of Glasgow Veterinary School
Bearsden Road
Bearsden Glasgow G61 1QH
Tel: (+44) 141 330 5705
Fax: (+44) 141 942 7215
Email: J.Wason@vet.gla.ac.uk

As one of the world's top 100 universities, the University of Glasgow combines tradition with academic excellence.

The school is one of only five veterinary schools in Europe to be accredited to British, European and American standards.

Building on more than 140 years of expertise, the School of Veterinary Medicine is at one and the same time a hospital, a research institute and a top-rated teaching establishment, training the next generation of veterinary practitioners and scientists.

It is in a unique position as the only Veterinary School in the UK where all the academic departments are located together. The single site houses preclinical and clinical departments, a small animal hospital and the Weipers Centre for Equine Welfare. Cochno Farm & Research Centre, an additional teaching facility, lies just five miles away.

The school has always taken great pride in its innovative teaching programmes and was the first in the UK to establish a totally clinical final year that helps to prepare students thoroughly for the world of work. Teaching is rated as 'excellent' by the latest independent Quality Assessment of Teaching. The school also achieved the highest results among all UK AVMA accredited schools for student satisfaction in the National Student Survey.

2009 saw the completion of a new state of the art £15m Small Animal Hospital and a new £2.5m production animal facility. The current hospital treats over 9,000 cases each year and the number is growing steadily. It provides a referral service to veterinary general practitioners and its staff includes clinicians for all specialities.

The city of Glasgow has a population of around 74,000 and is Scotland's largest city. One of Europe's liveliest places with a varied and colorful cultural and social life, it can cater to every taste. Situated on the River Clyde, Glasgow has excellent road and rail links to the rest of the UK and air services to a wide range of destinations, both home and overseas.

Wherever you come from, you can be sure of building friendships that last a lifetime at Glasgow. According to travel guide Lonely Planet, Glasgow is one of the world's top ten cities.

Application Information

For specific application information (availability, deadlines, fees, and VMCAS participation), please refer to the contact information listed above.

Residency implications: Due to recent changes in immigration legislation, students from the U.S. (who are planning to come to the UK for more than 6 months) are now required to obtain an entry clearance certificate prior to entering the UK. For further information on entry to the UK, please refer to http://www.ukvisas.gov.uk. Students must also be able to ensure adequate financial support for the duration of their course.

Prerequisites for Admission

Course requirements
3 years of full-time university study; subjects to include organic chemistry, biology, math, and (if possible) a knowledge of physics and a cumulative average of around 70%.

Required undergraduate GPA: 3.40.

AP credit policy: not applicable.

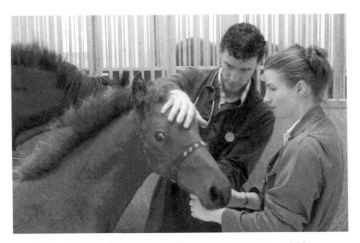

The Equine Centre for Equine Welfare at the University of Glasgow Veterinary School offers state-of-the-art technology to children's ponies and to Cheltenham winners alike. Photo courtesy of Joyce Wason, University of Glasgow Veterinary School.

Course completion deadline: required courses should be completed prior to admission in the fall.

Standardized examinations: none required. GRE® results will be considered if submitted.

Additional requirements and considerations
    Animal/veterinary work experience sufficient to indicate motivation, interest, and understanding of the veterinary profession
    Evaluations: minimum 2, one each from an academic science source and a veterinary surgeon.

Summary of Admission Procedure

Timetable
    VMCAS application deadline: Friday, October 1, 2010 12:00 PM (noon) Eastern Time
    Date interviews held: February–March (in the U.S.)
    Date acceptances mailed: April
    School begins: late September

Deposit (to hold place in class): $2,500

Deferments: in certain circumstances.

Evaluation criteria
    Academic performance
    Animal/veterinary experience
    References
    Essay
    Interview

2008–2009 admissions summary

	Number of Applicants	Number of New Entrants
In-province	1,100	72
International	350	50
Total:	1,450	122

Expenses for entry in 2011

Tuition and fees
    Resident   residents of the UK are government-funded
    International   £21,000

For further information, contact Joyce Wason (J.Wason@vet.gla.ac.uk).

University of Guelph

Admissions, Office of Registrarial Services
University Centre, Level 3
University of Guelph
Guelph Ontario N1G 2W1
Canada
Telephone: (519) 824-4120, ext. 56062
www.ovc.uoguelph.ca

Founded in 1862, the Ontario Veterinary College is located in Guelph, Ontario. About 97 miles north of Buffalo. Guelph has a similar climate to Detroit and Chicago. Surrounded by gently rolling farmland and known for its safety, friendly people, warm summers and brisk winters, this city of 126,000 is typical of the northeast.

The university has an enrollment of over 19,000 undergraduate students of which 440 are in the Doctor of Veterinary Medicine (DVM) program. There are also approximately 200 graduate students, 100 faculty and 200 staff members at the veterinary college, which offers degree programs leading to a DVM, MPH, MSc, PhD, Doctor of Veterinary Science (DVSc) and a Graduate Diploma. The college has 4 departments: Population Medicine, Clinical Studies, Biomedical Sciences; and Pathobiology with 10 million $C in research funding from various government and private sector sources. The site features a full-service teaching hospital with both a large animal and a small animal clinic. There are also large, modern research stations for separately housing sheep, swine, and dairy and beef cattle, and a Centre for Public Health and Zoonoses. In 2010 we will be opening our new Hill's Pet Nutrition Primary Healthcare Centre, a unique educational centre ensuring OVC will continue to be an international leader in learning, teaching and research in companion animal primary health care and service delivery.

Application Information

For specific application information (availability, deadlines, fees, and VMCAS participation), please refer to the contact information listed above.

Residency implications: International applicants will be considered provided the applicant does not hold Canadian citizenship or permanent resident status in Canada. There is a maximum of 15 international positions available per year.

Prerequisites for Admission

Course requirements and semester hours: Students must first complete a minimum of two full-time years (four full-time semesters) of university including specific university courses. Students initially apply for admission to a science degree program. For the purpose of DVM admission, a full-time semester will include at least 5 one-semester courses. Once the prerequisite courses are completed successfully, students apply for admission to the DVM Program. The subject matter requirements listed below must have been completed before admission to the DVM program will be considered.

Course requirements and semesters

Biological sciences (emphasis on animal biology; one semester must be cell biology)	3
Genetics	1
Biochemistry	1
Statistics (with a university-level calculus prerequisite)	1
Humanities or social sciences*	2

* Students entering the DVM program should be able to operate across discipline boundaries recognizing the relevance of the humanities and social sciences to their career choice. In selecting these courses from among those acceptable, the prospective veterinary student should consider topics such as ethics, logic, critical thinking, determinants of human behavior, and human social interaction.

Required courses proposed to be completed at an institution other than the University of Guelph should be approved as acceptable prior to registration. Applicants are required to request approval for courses in writing. Course descriptions must be included with the request. Courses will not be acceptable if they are repeats of previously passed courses, or if they are taken at the same or a lower level in a subject area than previously passed courses in the same subject area. It is expected that the required undergraduate preparation for the DVM program will be completed in a full-time coherent academic program.

Required undergraduate GPA: students with a minimum GPA of 3.00 on a 4.00 scale based on the average of the required courses and the last 2 semesters in full-time attendance at university may be further considered.

Course completion deadline: required courses must be completed by December 31 of the year prior to application in order to be further considered.

Standardized examinations: Non-Canadian applicants submit Graduate Record Examination (GRE) scores. The code for GRE scores is 0892. For Canadian applicants Medical College Admission Test (MCAT) is required. Test scores must be received no later than December 1 of the year of application.

Additional requirements and considerations

Reasons for choosing a career in veterinary medicine
Quality of preparatory academic program

Experience and knowledge in matters relating to animals and to the
veterinary medical profession
Experience and achievement in extracurricular affairs and/or
community service activities
Communication skills
Referees' reports

Summary of Admission Procedure

Timetable
VMCAS application deadline: Friday, October 1, 2010 12:00 PM
(noon) Eastern Time; December 1 for all others
Date interviews are held: February–May
Date acceptances mailed: March–July
School begins: September

Deposit (to hold place in class): A non-refundable deposit of $1,500.00 Cdn is
due after an offer of acceptance is made to hold a seat in the class.

2008–2009 admissions summary

	Number of Applicants	Number of New Entrants
Residents	251	105
International Residents	85	15
Total:	336	120

Expenses for the 2008–2009 Academic Year

Tuition and fees
Resident	$6,961.12 $C
Visa student	$53,945.12 $C

Massey University

International Student Affairs
Massey University Vet School
Institute of Veterinary, Animal and Biomedical Sciences
College of Sciences
Massey University
Private Bag 11-222
Palmerston North
New Zealand
Tel: (+646) 350 4473
Fax (+646) 350 5699
Email: vetschool@massey.ac.nz
http://vet-school.massey.ac.nz/

Massey University is located "down under" in picturesque New Zealand. The vet school is located in Palmerston North, a student-friendly town of 75,000 in the lower central north island of New Zealand. Nicknamed "student city," Palmerston North offers free bus service and free bikes to Massey students and is home to numerous cafés, restaurants, bars, theatres, and outdoor recreational activities. Palmerston North is a one-hour flight from Auckland and just under a two-hour drive to Wellington City and the ski fields of Mt. Ruapehu.

The Massey University Veterinary School accepts up to 24 international students annually with a total class size of just under 100. The first class of Massey veterinarians graduated in 1967, and since then more than 2,500 veterinarians have graduated and are working around the world.

The Massey University veterinary program has an international reputation for providing an excellent veterinary education with a strong science background, a broad knowledge of companion, equine, and production animal health, and a focus on independent thinking and problem-solving skills. The curriculum incorporates practical aspects throughout all years of the degree beginning with animal handling and behaviour in the first post-selection semester through to the final year of the program, which is almost entirely clinically based.

The veterinary facilities are of a high international standard with numerous other university-run animal units (farms, equine blood typing unit, feline unit, large animal teaching unit, etc.) on or adjacent to the Palmerston North campus. The veterinary teaching hospital sees first-opinion cases as well as referral cases to provide a balanced clinical experience for the students. The Massey University veterinary college staff are collegial, motivated, highly qualified individuals, many of whom have trained in the United States or are board certified specialists in their discipline.

Studying in New Zealand will give you the opportunity to see some of the world while studying toward your veterinary qualification and broadening your perspectives in life.

Application Information

For specific information (availability, deadlines, fees, and VMCAS participation), please refer to the contact information listed above.

Residency implications: All non-New Zealand residents require a student visa, which is easily obtained following an offer of admission into the program. Students must be able to ensure financial support for the duration of their course.

Prerequisites for Admissions

Course requirements

Group 1—Competitive Selection into Vet School via Semester 1 (10-14 places available)
Group 1 applicants are required to come to Massey University and complete a semester (beginning in late February of each year) of full-time study (4 classes) at Massey University in order to develop a GPA for selection. Credit will be given where similar classes to the four prerequisite classes have already been completed, and other classes will be taken in their place.

Group 2—Competitive Selection directly into BVSc Semester 2 (10-14 places available)
Applicants are required to have completed at least two full years of full-time, largely science based university education. Applicants need to have passed classes equivalent to the 4 standard Massey University veterinary prerequisite classes:

Massey University Class	Usual classes needed for credit
Chemistry and Living Systems	General chemistry + Organic chemistry
Physics for Life Sciences	1 year of physics
Biology of Cells	Cell (molecular) biology +/– Genetics
Biology of Animals	Animal biology / organismal zoology

Each of the above classes should include laboratories.

Required undergraduate GPA: a minimum science GPA of 3.00 is required to be eligible for selection into the veterinary degree.

Course completion deadline:
> Group 2: all required courses should be completed by the end of the fall
> semester in the year prior to matriculation.
> Group 1: not applicable; courses completed in New Zealand.

Standardized examinations: Graduate Record Examination (GRE®), general test, is required for Group 2 applicants only. The minimum GRE score required is 1600 for all 3 sections (this may be subject to change). The analytical written score out of 6 is converted to a score out of 800 and added to the verbal and quantitative scores. Test scores can be no older than 5 years immediately preceding the application deadline. Score must be received by the application deadline (see below).

Additional requirements and considerations:
A letter signed by a veterinarian on his/her clinic letterhead verifying a minimum of 10 days' work experience at the clinic completed by the applicant.

A bachelor's degree is not a prerequisite requirement for admission into the veterinary degree.

Summary of Admission Procedure

Timetable
> Group 1 (semester 1)
>> Application deadline: December 1
>> Date letters of admission to semester 1 sent: once completed
>> application received and processed.
>> School begins: late February (semester 1)
>> Date acceptances into the veterinary degree program mailed: early July
>> Date veterinary degree program begins: mid-July (semester 2)
> Group 2
>> VMCAS application deadline: Friday, October 1, 2010 12:00 PM
>> (noon) Eastern Time (VMCAS application completed online.
>> Supplemental application with all supplementary documents to be
>> received by October 15.)
>> Direct applicants: October 15 (including all supplementary documents)
>> Date acceptances mailed: from late December
>> School begins: mid-July (semester 2)

Deposit (to hold Group 2 position): $NZ 5,000.00

Deferments: offers of a place in semester 2 of the program are for a single year only. Deferments are not permitted. Deferments of offers of a place in semester 1 of the program (Group 1 applicants) are permitted.

Evaluation criteria
    Group 1
        Weighted GPA   80%
            (Minimum of a B average across all 4 first semester
            classes needed to be considered for selection).
        Special Tertiary Admissions Test (STAT)   20%
            This is the Australian equivalent to the GRE®
            and is held at Massey University at the end of the
            first semester.
        Top 10-14 applicants offered places
    Group 2
        Science GPA   50%
        GRE® General Test   50%
        Students will be offered places in order of their ranking until 10-14
            places are filled.

2008 admissions summary

	Number of Applicants	*Number of New Entrants*
Residents	275	75
International		
Group 1	45	22
Group 2	<u>105</u>	<u>2</u>
Total:	425	99

Expenses for the 2010 Academic Year

Tuition

Resident	residents of New Zealand are government-subsidised	
International	Semester 1	$NZ 11,200
	Semesters 2–9	$NZ 23,250 ($NZ 46,500 per year)

The University of Melbourne

Admissions Office
The Faculty of Veterinary Science
The University of Melbourne
Corner Park Drive and Flemington Road
Parkville
3010
Melbourne
Victoria
Australia
Tel: + (613) 8344 7357
Fax: + (613) 8344 7374
Email: http://vet-unimelb.custhelp.com
www.vet.unimelb.edu.au

The University of Melbourne has a 150 year history of leadership in research, innovation, teaching and learning. As a University of Melbourne student, you will become part of a dynamic collegial environment with a distinctive research edge. Throughout its history the University of Melbourne has educated some of the world's most eminent scientists and researchers and this tradition continues today.

The Faculty of Veterinary Science was the very first veterinary school established in Australia, and celebrated its centenary in 2009. It is concentrated on two sites: the city-centre University campus in Parkville and the Werribee campus, where students study in a state-of-the-art teaching hospital designed to support top-class veterinary education in the 21st century. Facilities include ten consulting rooms, modern diagnostic capabilities including endoscopy, CT, MRI, image intensification, scintigraphy, on-site diagnostic pathology laboratories and a 24-hour small animal emergency and critical care unit.

The veterinary program is made up of industry-linked learning, practical components and internship opportunities. Students gain experience in animal handling, care and management and undertake professional work experience between semesters and academic years, as well as having hands-on experience throughout the course. The school has strong programs in equine, dairy cattle, sheep and beef cattle medicine.

The degree is accredited by the American Veterinary Medical Association (AVMA), by the Royal College of Veterinary Surgeons (UK), and by the Australasian Veterinary Boards Council Inc. These accreditations reflect the high quality and international standing of the course and permits graduates of the 151 course to work as veterinarians in a wide range of countries including North America.

Our success has been achieved by insisting on international excellence. Talented people from all over the world come to visit, study and work at the University of Melbourne. At last count, the University's student community of 44,000 included more than 9,800 international students from over 100 countries.

We invite you to join our tradition and discover why staff and students of the highest calibre are attracted to study at the Faculty of Veterinary Science at the University of Melbourne.

Course duration, entry routes and student numbers

Please note that as from 2011 we will be moving to a new model of education; the Melbourne Model. We will continue to offer exceptional veterinary education through our newly created professional entry graduate degree; the Doctor of Veterinary Medicine*. The new four-year degree will offer veterinary students the best possible preparation for twenty-first century careers in a rapidly changing and increasingly global workforce. As a result of this change, students can enter the veterinary science program by one of two pathways:

1. Students can apply for entry into the three-year Bachelor of Science degree at the University of Melbourne. After completing prerequisite first and second year subjects, students will apply for selection to the Veterinary Bioscience specialisation that will be offered in the third year of the Bachelor of Science. Students who successfully complete all studies in the Veterinary Bioscience specialisation will have guaranteed entry to the DVM* program with 100 points' credit (one year of DVM* study).
2. Students can also complete a science degree at the University of Melbourne or another institution, and then apply for entry to the DVM* at the University of Melbourne. Students will need to have studied at least one semester in each of general or cellular biology and biochemistry within their science degree. Students who follow this pathway will enter the four-year graduate-entry DVM* program, which will be available at the University of Melbourne from 2011.

Number of international students that we accept

We currently accept up to 50 international students from across the globe.

Prerequisites for Admissions

1. Entrance to the DVM via the Melbourne Bachelor of Science: North American students should refer to the University's international prospectus for up to date details about entrance requirements for the Bachelor of Science by visiting http://www.futurestudents.unimelb. edu.au/publications

151

After completing prerequisite first and second year subjects in the Bachelor of Science, students will be eligible to apply for entry to the Veterinary Bioscience specialisation in third year. Students who successfully complete all studies in the Veterinary Bioscience specialisation will have guaranteed entry into the DVM, with 100 points' credit (one year of study), leaving three years of study in the DVM.

2. Entrance to the DVM as a graduate: Applicants will require a science degree from the University of Melbourne or another institution. Examples of appropriate degrees include Bachelor's degrees with majors in: Agriculture, Animal Science, Biochemistry, Biomedicine, Physiology or Zoology. Prerequisites for entry as a graduate are at least one semester of study in each of general or cellular biology and biochemistry as part of a science degree.

Application Information

International applications will be accepted throughout the course of the year. Applications will be considered as soon as they are received. We recognise the amount of time required by successful applicants in order to make arrangements for international travel and study and we try to give them as much advance notice as possible.

Students apply via the International Admissions Office at the University of Melbourne. They can choose to apply online, download an application form, apply through one of our overseas representatives or request an undergraduate application form to be posted to them. Visit http://www.futurestudents.unimelb.edu.au/int for further information.

Application fee: AUD$100.

Visas: All non-Australian students require a student visa, which is easily obtained following an offer of admission into our program. More information can be viewed on the web site—www.services.unimelb.edu.au/international/visas.

Deferments: Please note that successful applicants may not apply to defer commencement of the new DVM*. Students can reapply, and the application fee will be waived for international students.

For more specific information including fee information please refer to the contact information listed above.

*pending Academic Board approval

Université de Montréal

Service de l'admission et du recrutement
Université de Montréal
C.P. 6205
Succursale Centre-Ville
Montréal Québec H3C 3T5
Canada
Téléphone: (514) 343-7076
Email: saefmv@medvet.umontreal.ca
www.medvet.umontreal.ca

Renseignements pour les demandes d'admission/Application Information

Formulaires disponibles dès: décembre
    En Ligne: 80 $
    Papier: 100 $

Applications available: December
    On line: 80 $
    Paper: 100 $

Date limite de remise: 1ᵉʳ février

Application deadline: February 1

Statut de résident: Il faut être citoyen canadien ou résident permanent pour être admissible.

Residency implications: Canadian citizenship or permanent residency in Canada is required.

Prérequis/Prerequisites for Admission

DEC (Diplôme d'Etudes Collégiales) incluant les cours suivants:

Cours/Course requirements
Physique/Physics	101, 201, 301–78
Chimie/Chemistry	101, 201, 202
Biologie/Biology	301, 401
Mathématiques (avec calcul intégral)/ Mathematics (including calculus)	103, 203

Pour être admis au programme de DMV, il faut: a) avoir satisfait les conditions ci-dessus, ou b) faire preuve d'études équivalentes.

To be considered for admission, one must: a) have completed the above requirements, or b) have completed equivalent studies.

Note: All lectures are given in French. Examinations must be written in French.

Le programme de DMV est réparti sur cinq ans.

The DMV is a 5-year program.

Condition relative à la langue française: pour être admissible, le candidat doit attester d'une connaissance de la langue française atteignant le degré que l'Université estime minimal pour s'engager dans le programme. À cette fin, il doit:

- soit avoir réussi l'Épreuve uniforme de langue et littérature française du ministère de l'Éducation du Québec;
- soit obtenir un score d'au moins 785/990 au Test de français international (TFI) http ://www.etudes.umontreal.ca/programme/doc_prog/section2.pdf.

Condition concerning the knowledge of French: To be admissible, the candidate must demonstrate that he/she has acquired the minimal level of proficiency in French as required by the chosen program, as established by the University. To this end, the candidate must either:

- succeed the Épreuve uniforme de langue et littérature française of the Ministry of Education of Quebec or;
- obtain a score of at least 785/990 on the International French exam (Test de français international TFI) http://www.etudes.umontreal.ca/programme/doc_prog/section2.pdf.

Performance Score: This score is obtained by comparing the student's grade in each course with the class average.

Dossier académique avant admission: Le candidat doit, ou bien avoir terminé, tous les cours préalables au moment de la demande d'admission.

Course completion deadline: The applicant must have completed all prerequisites at the time of application.

Critères de sélection (priorité d'importance)/Additional considerations (in order of importance)

1. Dossier académique
2. Entrevue: l'entrevue vise à évaluer les compétences transversales.

1. Academic record
2. Interview: the interview is designed to verify the transversal competencies.

Cédule du processus/Summary of Admission Procedure

Horaire

Date limite pour les demandes d'admission: le 1er février

Entrevues: début du mois de mai

Offres d'admission: fin mai, début juin
Début de l'année scolaire: fin août

Timetable
    Application deadline: February 1
    Interviews: beginning of May
    Notification of acceptance: end of May, early June
    Fall semester begins: end of August

Dépôt nécessaire pour garder une place dans la classe: 200 $C.
Deposit (to hold place in class): 200 $C.

Critères d'évaluation/Evaluation criteria	%
Résultats scolaires/Performance score	60
Entrevue/Interview	40

Budget estimé/Estimated Expenses for the 2009–2010 Academic Year

Frais de scolarité:	65.60 $C	par crédit pour les étudiants québécois (approx. 45 crédits par année)
Tuition and fees:	65.60 $C	per credit for residents of Quebec (approx. 45 per year)

183.36 $ par crédit pour les étudiants canadiens non-residents du
    Québec
183.36 $ per credit for canadians non-residents of Quebec

Murdoch University

Murdoch International
Murdoch University
South Street
Murdoch 6150
Western Australia
Tel: (61-8) 9360 6770
Fax: (61-8) 9310 5090
Email: internat@murdoch.edu.au
http://www.vetbiomed.murdoch.edu.au/

Western Australia is known for its brilliant blue skies, warm sunny climate and white sandy beaches. It is a land blessed with some of the world's most precious natural phenomena including the dolphins of Monkey Mia, the 350-million-year-old Bungle Bungle range and the towering karri forests of the South West. Sophisticated yet uncomplicated, the lifestyle for the residents of Perth is relaxed and focuses on the outdoors. There are wineries, beaches and bushland within easy reach of the city, and a cosmopolitan mix of cafes, restaurants, pubs and thriving nightlife in the city centre.

Veterinary Science is a five year double degree (Bachelor of Science and Bachelor of Veterinary Medicine and Surgery) designed to impart the knowledge and skills necessary for the diagnosis, treatment and prevention of disease and production problems in pets, farm animals, wildlife and laboratory animals. Veterinary students learn in a true practice atmosphere with the final year of study lecture-free and devoted entirely to clinical exposure, including time spent at Perth Zoo and the Western Australian Department of Agriculture in Albany. Murdoch students have access to state-of-the art facilities, all on the one campus, including a 24-hour emergency clinic, the large and small animal practices, a well-stocked farm and an equine hospital.

A new curriculum that commenced in 2008 keeps Murdoch at the forefront of veterinary education worldwide. The new curriculum allows more time for students to develop areas of special interest through non-core rotations, special topics, externships and extramural experience. A Veterinary Professional Life stream is integrated throughout the course to assist students in their transition to future careers in veterinary science and provides a strong focus for developing professional life skills within the veterinary profession. An Animal Systems stream will allow strengthening and integration of animal production, animal ethics, animal welfare, animal behaviour, biosecurity and veterinary public health throughout the veterinary program.

The veterinary science degree is accredited by the American Veterinary Medical Association (AVMA), the Royal College of Veterinary Surgeons (UK), and the Australian Veterinary Boards Council.

Application Information

For specific information (availability, deadlines, fees, and VMCAS participation), please refer to the contact information listed above.

All non-residents require a student visa, which is easily obtained following an offer of admission into the veterinary course. Applicants whose first language is not English must demonstrate competency in the English language.

Admission Requirements

Murdoch University does not generally require completion of any prerequisite secondary subjects however, students would be best prepared for the courses if they have a background in Mathematics, Chemistry, and either Physics or Biology. Students will need to meet specific English competency requirements.

From 2008 the admission requirements have been altered to allow for more clinical experience to be built into the final years of studies. This means that students will have to complete one year or more of tertiary study to be eligible to enter the five year Veterinary course. Your first year of tertiary study must include units in Chemistry, Cell Function, and Statistics.

Applications are still accepted from school leavers, with high achievers offered a guaranteed place in the veterinary course, provided they pass their first year of tertiary study at Murdoch University.

Other applicants will be formally selected from those who have successfully completed one year or more of formal tertiary study, including the prerequisite units listed above. Applicants are required to supply with the application form a typed Personal Statement of up to 500 words to which should be attached documents such as curriculum vitae and references, and which should outline:

- why you wish to become a Veterinarian;
- how you consider your past study and experience to date will assist you to succeed in the veterinary course, and as a Veterinarian. If you have any fails/late withdrawals in your post-secondary/tertiary study, you should explain the circumstances for your poor performance and why those circumstances will not apply to your Murdoch studies. You should aim to demonstrate your motivation and preparation for veterinary science.

Assessment of the application will be based on the academic standard achieved in all previous tertiary study, the personal statement, and evidence of recent veterinary and related experience. Depending on whether an applicant has satisfied the prerequisites, an offer will be made directly into the veterinary course. If not, an offer will be made into another course with an assured progression into the veterinary course after successful completion of that year.

Summary of Admission Procedure

Timetable

There are four application deadlines each year, which are:
March 31, June 30, September 30 and November 30.
School begins: mid February.
Some candidates may be eligible to begin in early August.

VMCAS application deadline: Friday, October 1, 2010. 12:00 PM (noon) Eastern Time.

Deposit to hold a position: $1,000 AUD payable upon acceptance of offer

Expenses for the 2010 Academic Year

Tuition fees:
General Science first year A$23,000 pa
Veterinary Science A$39,950 pa

Deferments: not considered

University of Prince Edward Island

Registrar's Office
Atlantic Veterinary College
University of Prince Edward Island
550 University Avenue
Charlottetown PEI C1A 4P3
Canada
Telephone: (902) 566-0781
Email: registrar@upei.ca
www.upei.ca/registrar/

The Atlantic Veterinary College (AVC), one of the newest colleges of veterinary medicine in North America, opened in 1986 and is fully accredited by the American Veterinary Medical Association, the Canadian Veterinary Medical Association, and the Royal College of Veterinary Surgeons (UK).

Centrally located on Canada's eastern seaboard (650 miles northeast of Boston), the Atlantic Veterinary College makes its home in a beautiful island setting in Charlottetown, Prince Edward Island. With a population of 138,000, which jumps to over a million during the summer tourist season, the community enjoys a small-town lifestyle that boasts the amenities of larger cities, including dining and theatre. Residents also enjoy outdoor activities, such as golfing, cycling, sailing, and cross-country skiing.

The college is a completely integrated teaching, research, and service facility. The four-story complex contains the veterinary teaching hospital, diagnostic services, fish health unit, farm services, postmortem services, animal barns, laboratories, classrooms, computer and audio-visual facilities, offices, cafeteria, and study areas.

Prince Edward Island is a scenic province with a wide variety of dairy, beef, hog, sheep, horse, and fish farms. The combination and variety of animal and fish farms have allowed AVC to develop a special expertise in fish health, aquaculture, and population medicine.

Application Information

For specific application information (availability, deadlines, fees, and VMCAS participation), please refer to the contact information listed above.

Residency implications: Atlantic Veterinary College contracts with New Brunswick (13), Newfoundland (3), Nova Scotia (16), and the home province P.E.I. (10). International students are admitted on a noncontract basis (up to 21).

Prerequisites for Admission

The preveterinary program leading to admission at the Atlantic Veterinary College will normally be completed within the context of a 2-year science program.

Course requirements
Twenty 1-semester courses or equivalent are required. Normally, these courses must be completed while the applicant is enrolled as a full-time student carrying at least 3 courses per semester, at a minimum of 9 semester hours' credit excluding labs. Science courses will normally have a laboratory component and be completed within 6 years of the date of application. Exceptional circumstances will be given consideration; however, it is necessary for all applicants to demonstrate the ability to master difficult subject matter in the context of full-time activity.

Courses must include:

Mathematics	1 course
Statistics	1 course
Biological sciences	2 courses, with labs (emphasis on Animal Biology*)
Microbiology	1 course with lab
Genetics	1 course
Chemistry	3 courses with labs, one being Organic Chemistry
Physics	1 course with lab
English	2 courses, one being English Composition
Humanities and social sciences	3 courses
Electives	5 courses from any discipline

* Examples of animal biology courses include first-year general biology, vertebrate anatomy, vertebrate histology, vertebrate physiology, vertebrate zoology, molecular biology, and cell biology.

Applicants are encouraged to work towards an undergraduate degree. It is recommended that applicants consider including courses in the following topics in their preveterinary curriculum: personal finance, small business management, psychology, sociology, biochemistry, ethics, and logic.

Required undergraduate GPA: no minimum stated (under review as stated above); mean cumulative GPA of most recent entering class is 3.70 on a 4.00 scale.

AP and IB credit policy: a maximum of 6 credits accepted.

Course completion deadline: June 1 of the year of application.

Standardized examinations: Graduate Record Examination (GRE®)

If a student's native language or language of prior education is not English, then the student will be required to pass one of the following: TOEFL, MELAB, IELB, or CanTest.

Additional requirements and considerations
    Animal/veterinary experience
    Interview—assessing noncognitive skills
    Extracurricular activities

Summary of Admission Procedure

Timetable
    VMCAS application deadline: Friday, October 1, 2010 12:00 PM (noon)
        Eastern Time; November 1 for supplementary application; and
        January 1 for transfer
    Date interviews are held: February–March
    Date acceptances mailed: April
    School begins: late August; registration, early September

Deposit (to hold place in class): 500.00 $C

Deferments: are considered on a case-by-case basis.

Evaluation criteria
Academic credentials including the GRE are evaluated by the Registrar's Office. Other criteria and activities are evaluated by the admissions committee through an interview process, and the supplementary application.

	% weight
Academic ability	55
Noncognitive ability	35
Veterinary experience	10

2008–2009 admissions summary

	Number of Applicants	Number of New Entrants
In-Province	20	10
Contract*	86	32
International	269	21
Total:	375	63

* For further information, see the listing of contracting states and provinces.

Expenses for the 2009–2010 Academic Year

Tuition and fees
    Resident   10,364.00 $C
    Contract student*   10,364.00 $C
    International student   51,053.00 $C (48,500 $US est.)

* For further information, see the listing of contracting states and provinces.

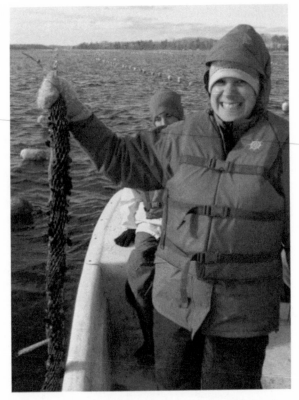

Photo courtesy of Atlantic Veterinary College, University of Prince Edward Island.

Royal Veterinary College

Margaret Kilyon
Head of Admissions
Royal Veterinary College
Royal College Street
London
NW1 0TU
Telephone: (+44) 20 7468 5146
Fax: (+44) 20 7468 5311
Email: international@rvc.ac.uk

The RVC has a successful record of training North American students and can count several hundred American graduates as alumni. Founded in 1791, the RVC was the first veterinary school in the UK, and the driving force behind the establishment of the nation's veterinary profession. The first four students were admitted in January 1792, and ever since the College has been at the forefront of teaching and research in the veterinary and allied sciences. The RVC was the first to submit a woman for membership to the Royal College of Veterinary Surgeons; become an independent veterinary school within a federal university; be accredited by the American Veterinary Medical Association; introduce a degree in Veterinary Nursing; offer a Masters programme in Veterinary Physiotherapy; and establish a Centre for Lifelong and Independent Veterinary Education. Today, first-class teaching and research staff, experienced in a wide range of disciplines and skills, help talented students to exploit state-of-the-art clinical facilities and laboratories to the full—maintaining the RVC's long, proud tradition of making seminal contributions to both the animal and human sciences.

We have one campus near Kings Cross/Camden Town, in central London (the London Campus) and one on the outskirts of London on a 575-acre site near Potters Bar (the Hertfordshire Campus). Both offer a friendly and supportive environment and excellent facilities for teaching and learning. The London Campus boasts newly refurbished research laboratories, an extensive library, an anatomy museum, the London Bioscience Innovation Centre and the Beaumont Animals' Hospital. Accommodation and a refectory are also on site and the clubs, bars, restaurants and theatres of Camden and London's West End are easily accessed on foot or by public transport. A twenty-minute walk from the London Campus is the University of London whose collegiate structure incorporates the RVC. Here in the capital's "university quarter," you will find some of the nation's greatest educational and research facilities. The Hertfordshire Campus is our main clinical campus with three state-of-the-art teaching hospitals on site including the largest veterinary-referral hospital in

Europe. Located in rural countryside near Potters Bar, it is a 20 minute train journey from London's King's Cross station and comprises lecture theatres, laboratories, a Learning Resources Centre, a Clinical Skills Centre and student housing. A refectory, playing fields, student bar and other leisure facilities mean the campus is quite self-contained. The Eclipse Building provides superb computer teaching and library facilities. In addition to its modern journals and textbooks, the RVC has one of the best collections of old veterinary books in the world.

Places in RVC halls of residence are available and students from overseas are given priority. The College has a number of dedicated staff who provide academic and pastoral support to students throughout the course, and we have an active and welcoming student community.

Application Information

For specific application information (availability, deadlines, fees and VMCAS participation), please refer to the contact information listed above.

Residency implications: The UK government introduced a points-based immigration system for students from non-EU countries who wish to study in the UK. For further information on entry to the UK, please refer to http:/www. ukvisas.gov.uk and to the College's web site. Students must also be able to ensure adequate financial support for the duration of their course.

Prerequisites for Admission

Course requirements
Applicants are normally final year or recent graduates although students with two years pre-vet will be considered. Science graduates or applicants in the final year of a science based degree with the prerequisites will be considered for our 4 year accelerated course. Applicants who are unsuccessful in gaining a place on the four year programme may be considered for our five year programme. Subjects must include Organic Chemistry with lab, Biochemistry, Mathematics or Statistics, Principles of Biology, Physics with lab, General Biology, Animal Biology, or Zoology all with lab. As a minimum we require 8 semester credits in Organic Chemistry and Principles of Biology, General Biology, Animal Biology or Zoology and 4 semester credits in Biochemistry, Physics with Laboratory and Mathematics/Statistics (including Algebra). It is also recommended that students take General Chemistry or Fundamentals of Chemistry.

Required undergraduate GPA: 3.40 preferred (on 4.0 point scale).

AP credit policy: not accepted.

Course completion deadline: all required courses should be completed by July of the year of admissions.

Standardized examinations: GRE General plus either GRE Biology, Biochemistry, or Chemistry

Additional requirements and considerations
Applicants are also expected to have gained relevant work experience of handling animals. This should, where possible, include not only work in veterinary practice but other animal establishments.

Summary of Admission Procedure

Timetable
> VMCAS application deadline: Friday, October 1, 2010 12:00 PM (noon) Eastern Time
> Date interviews are held: February/March (held in the U.S.). Some interviews may be held earlier
> Date acceptances mailed: March/April
> School begins: September

Deposit (to hold place in class): £1,000 sterling

Deferments: may be considered in exceptional circumstances.

Evaluation criteria
> Academic performance
> Tests
> Animal/veterinary experience
> Interview
> References/evaluations (minimum 2 required—one from academic science source and one from a veterinary surgeon)
> Personal statement

2008–2009 admissions summary (for entry in 2009)

	Number of Applicants	Number of New Entrants
In-province	930	127
International	387	33
Total:	1,317	160

* The Royal Veterinary College joined VMCAS in the admissions cycle 2007–2008.

Expenses for the 2010–2011 Academic Year*

Tuition and fees

Resident	residents of the UK are government-funded by loans
International	£19,320 sterling

* For up-to-date information on fees and all further information regarding admission to the College, please visit our website.

University of Calgary Faculty of Veterinary Medicine Admissions

University of Calgary Faculty of Veterinary Medicine Admissions
TRW 2D03, 3280 Hospital Drive NW
Calgary, AB T2N 4Z6
Telephone: 403.220.8699
Facsimile: 403.210.8121
Email: vet.admissions@ucalgary.ca
Application Deadline: January 10

Doctor of Veterinary Medicine

The University of Calgary Faculty of Veterinary Medicine (UCVM) offers a four-year professional degree leading to a Doctor of Veterinary Medicine (DVM). Completion of at least two years of post-secondary instruction at a recognized university or at a college providing university-equivalency in coursework is required prior to application to the DVM program.

Admissions

Enrolment in the DVM program at UCVM is currently limited to approximately 32 students who are Alberta residents. The Admissions Committee selects students for the program on the basis of academic and non-academic factors. Students are assessed academically on performance in their best 2 full undergraduate years and in the required courses. Applicants meeting the academic eligibility requirements are invited for an interview day where non-academic factors are assessed. At interview day, applicants are required to complete an on-site essay and participate in a series of interviews and other activities. Applicants must attend interview day at their own expense. There is no entrance exam or requirement to complete the MCAT or GRE exams.

The admissions process identifies applicants who will flourish in a DVM program that prepares students for all aspects of veterinary medicine. Consistent with the UCVM mandate, preference will be given to applicants who demonstrate an interest in pursuing careers in general veterinary practice that support rural development and sustainability, and careers in the areas of emphasis. There is no specific animal or veterinary-related experience required; however, demonstration and understanding of the veterinary profession and animal industries relevant to the applicant's career interests is expected.

Applicants will be notified of the Admissions Committee's decision in June.

Eligibility

At present, applicants must be Alberta residents, as defined by the following rules.

(a) The Residence of an applicant remains that of his/her parent(s) unless a new Residence has been established in accordance with clause (b);

(b) The Residence of an applicant shall be considered to be Alberta, if the applicant has last resided in Alberta for a period of twelve consecutive months (without including any period during which the applicant was attending a college or university) prior to enrolment on the first day of classes;

(c) A Canadian citizen who is resident outside Canada and intends to re-establish residence in Canada shall be considered a resident of the province or territory of Canada where he/she last resided for a period of twelve consecutive months before leaving Canada; and,

(d) A person who is a permanent resident as defined in the Immigration Act (Canada) shall be considered to be a resident of the province or territory where he or she first landed unless the person is considered to be a resident of another province or territory of Canada pursuant to clause (b).

The Faculty of Veterinary Medicine does not normally accept applications from students who have withdrawn, who have been required to withdraw, or who have been expelled from any school or college of veterinary medicine.

In selecting veterinary medicine students, no consideration shall be given to factors irrelevant to performance such as gender, race, or religion. Nor will the vocation of an applicant's parent, guardian, or spouse be a consideration in the selection process.

Minimum Academic Requirements

Normally, the minimum academic requirements for an applicant to receive consideration for an admissions interview are:

(a) Completion of, or in the final semester of completion of, at least two years of full time post-secondary instruction at a recognized university or at a college providing university-equivalency in coursework. A full academic year is defined as a minimum of 4 courses per semester and 2 complete semesters, September - May (16 half-course equivalents).

(b) Completion of, or in the final semester of completion of, the following ten required courses, with a minimum combined average of 2.7 (B- or its equivalent) and a passing grade in each course:

Biology:	Two introductory Biology courses
Genetics:	One introductory Genetics course
Ecology:	One introductory Ecology course
Chemistry:	Two introductory Chemistry courses
Organic Chemistry:	One introductory Organic Chemistry course

Biochemistry:	One introductory Biochemistry course
Mathematics:	One introductory Statistics course
English:	One introductory English course

(c) A minimum average of 3.00 (B, or its equivalent) over the best two full undergraduate years.

(d) Applicants who present required courses that have been taken greater than 10 years prior to the application date will not normally be considered for admission. Exceptions may be made for applicants who have continued to work or study in a health-sciences related field following completion of an undergraduate degree.

Applicants are advised to monitor the UCVM Website for any exceptions or changes to these requirements.

English Language Proficiency

English language proficiency must be demonstrated for all applicants for whom English is not their first language. English language proficiency can be demonstrated in one of the following ways:

(a) Completion of at least two full years within a degree program offered by an accredited university in a country which the University of Calgary recognizes as English language proficiency exempt.

(b) A minimum score of 92 on the internet based TOEFL (Test of English as a Foreign Language) and a minimum score of 50 on the Test of Spoken English (TSE); or a minimum score of 237 on the computer based TOEFL and a minimum score of 50 on the TSE; or a minimum score of 580 on the paper based TOEFL and a minimum score of 50 on the TSE.

Applications

Application forms for the Faculty of Veterinary Medicine are available on the website http://vet.ucalgary.ca/students/admission.html). Applications will be considered from those students meeting the residency, English and academic admission requirements. Applications are to be submitted to the UCVM Office of Admissions by January 10th. Two sets of official transcripts are required, one sent in by February 7th and the second should be sent as soon as final marks are available in the spring and no later than June 7th. Transcripts should be sent directly to the UCVM Admissions Office.

Completed application forms include the following: complete personal information; a signed statement verifying Alberta residency status and verifying completion of the academic requirements; tthree letters of reference (required by January 30th); post-secondary transcripts submitted by the appropriate academic institution; a statement of work experience; and a statement of major extra-curricular activities.

Registration

All successful applicants are required to forward $115.00 deposit within 15 working days of notification of admission. Failure to do so may result in the position being assigned to another applicant. Such deposits will be applied to the first year's fees. An applicant who accepts a position but later rescinds his or her acceptance will forfeit the entire $115.00 deposit.

Successful applicants are required to have or receive immunization for tetanus and rabies following admission.

Accuracy of Registration

The DVM program will register successful applicants and ongoing students into all required yearly courses. Payment of fees is the student's responsibility through the Online Student Centre via My UofC web portal. For more information refer to the "Payment of Fees or Notification of Financial Assistance" in the Registration section of this Calendar.

Deferrals

Students wishing to apply for deferral should make this request in a letter to the UCVM Admissions Office within 15 days of the date at the top of their acceptance letter. Deferrals will be considered for academic and/or non-academic reasons. Deferral requests for attending other veterinary schools will not be accepted. It is at the sole discretion of the Dean to grant or deny a deferral.

University of Saskatchewan-Western College of Veterinary Medicine

Admissions Office
Western College of Veterinary Medicine
52 Campus Drive
University of Saskatchewan
Saskatoon Saskatchewan S7N 5B4
Canada
Telephone: (306) 966-7454
www.usask.ca/wcvm

The Western College of Veterinary Medicine is located in the city of Saskatoon, which has a population of about 220,000 and is the major urban center in central Saskatchewan. The city is also the major commercial center for central and northern Saskatchewan and is served by 2 national airlines with direct connections to all major centers in Canada.

The Western College of Veterinary Medicine is one of the few veterinary colleges where all health sciences and agriculture are offered on the same campus. The college is devoted to undergraduate education and has a reputation in Canada and in the northwestern United States for educating veterinarians who are well-rounded in general veterinary medicine and have good practical backgrounds. It has one of the best field-service caseloads in North America.

Application Information

For specific application information (availability, deadlines, fees, and VMCAS participation), please refer to the contact information listed above.

Residency implications: students are selected for quota positions from Alberta, British Columbia, Manitoba, Saskatchewan, and the Yukon, Nunavut, and Northwest Territories. Special consideration is given to self-identified individuals of aboriginal origin. Residents of foreign countries are not considered.

Prerequisites for Admission

Course requirements and semester hours

English	6
Physics	6
Biology	6
Genetics	3

Introductory chemistry	6
Organic chemistry	3
Mathematics or statistics	6
Biochemistry	6
Microbiology	3
Electives	15

Required undergraduate GPA: a minimum cumulative average of 70% is required.

Course completion deadline: prerequisite courses must be completed by the time of entry into the program.

Standardized examinations: none required.

Additional requirements and considerations
    Animal/veterinary work experience, motivation, and knowledge
    Maturity
    Leadership
    Communication skills

Summary of Admission Procedure

Timetable
    Application deadline: January 3
    Date interviews are held: May–June
    Date acceptances mailed: on or before July 1
    School begins: late August

Deposit (to hold place in class): none required.

Deferments: not considered.

Evaluation criteria
The 3-part admission procedure consists of an assessment of academic ability, a personal interview, and an overall assessment of the application file.

	% *weight*
Grades	60
Interview*	30
Judgment	10

* Interview selection is based entirely on academic performance.

171

2009–2010 admissions summary

	Number of Applicants	Number of New Entrants
Resident	56	20
Contract[†]	225	56
Nonresident	4	1
Total:	285	77

Expenses for the 2009–2010 Academic Year

Tuition and fees
Resident	$7,439.42 $C
Nonresident	
Contract student[†]	$7,439.42 $C
Other nonresident-Canadian	$7,439.42 $C

† For further information, see the listing of contracting states and provinces.

University of Sydney

Faculty of Veterinary Science
JD Stewart building
University of Sydney
Sydney NSW 2006
Telephone: 02 9351 2441
Fax: 02 9351 3056
Email: vet.science@sydney.edu.au
Website: http://sydney.edu.au/vetscience

The University of Sydney, founded in 1850, is Australia's first university. Over the past 150 years, the University has built an international reputation for its outstanding teaching and as a centre of research excellence. It is one of the largest universities in Australia, with over 47,000 students, including 9,000 international students from more than 100 different countries. Famous for its sandstone buildings, lawns, courtyards and parklands setting the University of Sydney's main campus is spread across 72-hectares and features sports ovals, three sports centres, indoor and outdoor swimming pools, two major complexes devoted to student recreation and services, the famous Quadrangle and many other beautiful modern and historic buildings.

Located only ten minutes by bus from the heart of the Sydney business district, the main campus provides easy access to national and international companies based in the city and its surrounding suburbs.

The Faculty of Veterinary Science was established in 1910 and is the oldest continuing Faculty of its kind in Australia. The Faculty is an international leader in veterinary and animal education and research. The Faculty maintains teaching hospitals on both the Camperdown and Camden campuses, where students and veterinarians work together in a clinical teaching and learning environment. Referral and primary accession cases are seen at both sites, while the University Veterinary Teaching Hospital at Camden also provides veterinary services to farms in the region. A wide range of companion animals, farm animals, racing animals, exotic and native species are seen. Visiting specialists complement faculty specialists in most disciplines in providing an excellent learning environment for veterinary students.

The Faculty delivers inspirational and innovative student-centred teaching that leads to an acceptance of the need for life-long, evidence-based learning whilst also providing clinical and research excellence through creative, collaborative programs.

The Bachelor of Veterinary Science produces graduates with the knowledge and skills to pursue many career options as veterinary scientists participating in the care and welfare of animals. Completion of this five-year course ensures students have a wide knowledge of the principles associated with every aspect of health and disease in animals – domestic and native.

Application Information

All international applicants must apply directly to the University of Sydney International Office. Application forms are available from the International Office website at http:// sydney.edu.au/internationaloffice/

Admission Requirements

Academic Performance: International students must have achieved a similar standard to that expected of an Australian student seeking entry. Applicants will be assessed on the basis of their academic achievement in their final year of secondary education (Year 12 or equivalent) or their tertiary studies as appropriate, from a recognized University. Minimum GPA required 2.80 on a 4.00 scale, however, applicants must demonstrate and aptitude for the sciences.

Standardized examinations: International Student Admission Test (ISAT) http://www.acer.edu.au/isat (Applicants may submit GRE scores in lieu of ISAT scores.)

Additional requirements and considerations: Applicants are also expected to have gained relevant work experience and animal handling. This should be demonstrated on the "Commitment to Veterinary Science" form that can be downloaded from the faculty web site http://sydney.edu.au/vetscience/future_students/

Prerequisites

Admission is based on a level of assumed knowledge, comprising Higher School Certificate (HSC) (or equivalent) mathematics, physics and chemistry, with biology as a distinct advantage. Prospective students who have not reached this level in these subjects will be permitted to enrol but must be aware of the need to undertake supplementary work to avoid placing themselves at a disadvantage.

Practical Experience

During the inter-semester and intra-semester breaks in Year 3 students are required to gain practical experience in animal husbandry. The fifth and final year is lecture free with students participating in practice-based activities and the management and care of patients.

Professional Recognition

Graduates of the BVSc are immediately eligible for registration for practice by all Australian state and territory veterinary surgeons' boards and are recognised by the Royal College of Veterinary Surgeons in the United Kingdom and the American Veterinary Medical Association.

Additional Information

There is a quota of approximately 35 places in first year for international students each year. Admission into the course is very competitive. You should have an interest and competence in basic science subjects, as well as an interest in the health and welfare of animals. You should be prepared for long hours of work.

Intending students are advised to seek work experience in veterinary practices and the animal industries.

Tuition Fees 2010

The tuition fee for year 1 International Students in 2010 is AUD$42,240.
Fees are indexed annually.

Utrecht University

Office for International Cooperation
Faculty of Veterinary Medicine
Utrecht University
Yalelaan 1
3584 CL Utrecht
The Netherlands
Telephone: +31.30.2532116
Email: bic@vet.uu.nl
www.uu.nl/dgk

Short history

In 1821 a state veterinary school was founded in Utrecht. Almost a century later, in 1918, the school acquired the status of an institution of higher learning and in 1925 it was incorporated into the State University of Utrecht and thereby became the first and until to date the only Faculty of Veterinary Medicine in the Netherlands. Utrecht University, founded in 1636, is one of the 14 universities in the Netherlands. The faculty of Veterinary Medicine is now one of the 6 faculties of Utrecht University. From 1961 onwards parts of Utrecht University were moved to a new campus site (De Uithof) just outside the city of Utrecht. In 1967 the first parts of the veterinary faculty were transferred. After 21 years, in 1988, the whole Faculty was reunited at this new location. In 2010 the reconstruction and rebuilding program of the veterinary clinics will be concluded. The Faculty of Veterinary Medicine is housed in modern and spacious buildings on a total surface of 60.000 m).

Organisation and staff

The faculty encompasses 8 departments with specialized facilities, a Faculty Office and a number of general services (e.g. leaning environment with audio-visual units and the library, pharmacy, experimental farms, slaughterhouse, museum, student computer rooms etc). In 2003 a major reconstruction process in the clinical departments started; most of these reconstructions have been completed. The faculty has an academic staff of 418 fte, including 32 full professors and an administrative and support staff of 484 fte. Most staff members can communicate well in English and most lecturers have experience in teaching veterinary medicine in the English language.

Undergraduate veterinary education

Admission of students to the 6-year undergraduate veterinary training programme (taught in Dutch) is limited to 225 each year, resulting in a total of 1400 students. They pass full examinations at the completion of the first year ('propaedeutisch' examination), the fourth year ('doctoraal' examination) and the sixth year ('dierenarts') examination or Doctor of Veterinary Medicine, DVM. In September 2007 the veterinary education under a Bachelor - Master (3+3 years) structure started with the 1st year of the bachelor programme. In 2010 the master education in veterinary medicine will start under the responsibility of the Academic School of the faculty.

Research and postgraduate education

Research at the faculty of Veterinary Medicine is the responsibility of the Institute for Veterinary Research (IVR). Research which is conducted as part of the postgraduate master programmes and PhD programme is linked to one of the research programmes of the IVR. The postgraduate master programmes were initiated from 1994 onwards. In 2007 the postgraduate master education became part of the Academic School and the four master programmes are integrated in the postgraduate educational Master of Science programme Veterinary Science from September 2008.

Quality of education

The faculty of Veterinary Medicine is accredited by the American Veterinary Medical Association (AVMA) and Canadian Veterinary Medical Association (CVMA) since 1973, the European Association of Establishments of Veterinary Education and the Dutch and Flemish Accreditation Organization.

Information about the admission to the Faculty of Veterinary Medicine for foreign students

In general foreign students who want to be admitted to a Dutch university need to have permission of the Board of Governors of the university they intend to go to.

Special rules apply for the study of Veterinary Medicine. The Dutch Ministry of Education has declared the so-called *numerus fixus* applicable to the study of Veterinary Medicine. This entails that only a limited amount of students is admitted each year. The number of admission- requests largely exceeds the number of allocations. Those restrictions affect both Dutch and foreign students. The available places are assigned by selection through interviews or drawing lots.

Application and Drawing Lots

Each year the minister of Education and Science lays down the number of students that can be admitted to the study of Veterinary Medicine. At this moment the number is 225. In order to take part in the lottery for placement, you need to complete an application form via Internet (start with web-site: www.uu.nl) and send this in before May 15th.

177

If you do not enroll you cannot participate in drawing lots. Without drawing a place by lot, admission to the study of Veterinary Medicine is ruled out.

Foreign diplomas

Foreign diplomas have to be evaluated and compared with the Dutch equivalent diplomas. This evaluation takes time and can result in the fact that you have to take supplementary exams before being accepted for the lottery.

Information about the evaluation of your diplomas can be obtained at:

Universiteit Utrecht, Admissions Office
P.O. Box 80 125, 3508 TC Utrecht, the Netherlands
Phone: +31 30 253 7000
Visiting Address: Leuvenlaan 19, Utrecht – De Uithof

Dutch Language Exam

If the result of the lottery is favorable, then - prior to admission to the study of Veterinary Medicine - you have to prove your (sufficient) knowledge of the Dutch language. This is a requirement under the Dutch law because the education is in the Dutch language. The owner of a foreign diploma therefore has to pass the exam "Dutch as Second Language program 2" (*Staatsexamen Nederlands als Tweede Taal, programma* 2) before being admitted.

Request information about language courses and the examinations at:

James Boswell Institute
P.O. Box 80148, 3508 TC Utrecht, The Netherlands
Phone: +31 30 253 8666

Tuition fees and scholarships

The tuition fee depends on your nationality and the programme you register for:

Nationality	Programme	Tuition 2010-2011
EU / EEA	All Bachelor's programmes	€1,672
Non EU / EEA	Arts, Humanities, Economics	€6,000
	Science or Biomedical	€9,200
	Medicine or Veterinary Medicine	€10,200

No financial aid is offered to foreign students. Neither the government nor the university grants scholarships to foreign students.

Residence Permit

Every foreign student who wants to receive academic education in the Netherlands needs a residence permit. More information can be obtained at the Admissions Office.

Supplementary exams are imposed prior to a possible admission; there is a 12 months period of preparation time from the date of arrival in the Netherlands. During this period you have to pass the exams; prolongation is not an option.

Additionally you have to be able to demonstrate that you have sufficient financial means. The Admissions Office will ask to give proof of an annual disposal of ca. €8.000,-

Documentation

When requesting admission, the following pieces of documentation have to be sent to the Admissions Office (see above):

- a short and concise curriculum vitae with a complete overview of the education
- a certified copy of the birth register
- certified copies of diplomas, subject overview, list of marks of secondary and (pre-) university education in Dutch, French, German, or English
- a copy of personal details from the passport

For further information about the admission to the study of Veterinary Medicine please contact:

Student advisor
Faculty of Veterinary Medicine
Department of Student Affairs
PO Box 80 163, 3508 TD Utrecht, the Netherlands
e-mail: osz@vet.uu.nl

AAVMC Affiliate Member Veterinary Medical Schools

NATIONAL AUTONOMOUS UNIVERSITY OF MEXICO (UNAM) COLLEGE OF VETERINARY MEDICINE

Office of Undergraduate Studies (División de Estudios Profesionales)
College of Veterinary Medicine (FMVZ)
Av. Universidad 3000
Circuito Interior
Delegación Coyoacán
México D.F. 04510
Telephone: 56 22 58 80
Email: www.fmvz.unam.mx
http://escolar.fmvz.unam.mx

The College of Veterinary Medicine is located in the south of the main UNAM campus of Mexico City's metropolitan area.

Application Information

Undergraduate admission of new students to the National Autonomous University of Mexico (UNAM) is done through the General Administration School Direction (DGAE).

In relation to the College of Veterinary Medicine, students are evaluated in terms of their general academic background, with emphasis paid on Biology, Chemistry, Physics and Mathematics.

There are two annual applications dates, in January and May. Information can be reviewed at www.escolar.unam.mx

Application forms can be found at the same web direction.

Residency implications: There are no resident implications. As everybody, the students have to do the admission test.

Prerequisites for Admission

Applicants must have at least a high school average grade of 70 %.

For students from foreign high schools, apart from the admission test, they have to submit all necessary official documents to Dirección General de Incorporación y Revalidación de Estudios (DGIRE) UNAM. Submission instructions can be found at http://www.dgire.unam.mx/contenido/revalidacion/revalbachc.html.

Foreign students whose primary language is not Spanish will have to do a proficiency Spanish language test.

Required undergraduate GPA: It is not necessary

AP credit policy: Is not part of the admission requirements

Course completion deadline: It is based on the application dates, in January and May.

Standardized Examinations: They are not used

Additional requirements and considerations: Foreign students must have a good command of the Spanish language

Summary of Admission Procedure

Timetable
> The next application date is May 3, 2010. It can be checked at www.escolar.unam.mx

Deposit: It is not necessary

Deferments: Considered on an individual basis, and ordinarily granted for personal reasons, illness, lack of economic resources or other situations beyond the control of the students.

Evaluation criteria: Grade of 80% or above in the admission exam.

2009–2010 admissions summary

Number of Applicants	Number of New Entrants
2,169	130 (5.9%)

Expenses for the 2008–2009 Academic Year (subject to change)

Tuition and fees
> $2,000 USD per year

Dual-Degree Program

Does not apply

Leadership Program

Does not apply

Ross University School of Veterinary Medicine

Office of Admissions
Ross University School of Veterinary Medicine
630 US Highway 1
North Brunswick, NJ 08902
Toll-free telephone: 1-877-ROSS-EDU
Fax: 732-509-4803
Email: Admissions@RossU.edu
www.RossU.edu

Since its founding in 1982, Ross University School of Veterinary Medicine has graduated more than 2,400 veterinarians. The University maintains a technologically advanced campus in St. Kitts, which is located approximately 220 miles southeast of San Juan, Puerto Rico. St. Kitts is a beautiful island with large natural beaches, coral gardens, quaint villages, mountain gorges and rainforests. Together with her sister island, Nevis, they constitute the Federation of St. Christopher and Nevis, which is an English-speaking member of the British Commonwealth of Nations. Until recently, St. Kitts and Nevis were primarily agricultural, with sugar cane as the main crop. Economic growth is beginning to bring the islands into the mainstream of the tourism industry, and they are becoming known as pleasant and comfortable vacation destinations.

The seven-semester pre-clinical curriculum is enhanced by hands-on clinical experience to help prepare students for the final year of clinical training at one of Ross' affiliated veterinary schools in the United States. The University's faculty have outstanding credentials in teaching and research and share a passion for educating the veterinarians of tomorrow. Ross University operates on a three-semester per year calendar.

Each semester is 15 full academic weeks, including final exams. The University is affiliated with 22 American Veterinary Medical Association (AVMA)-accredited schools of veterinary medicine where students complete their clinical training. Ross University graduates are eligible to practice veterinary medicine in all 50 States, Canada and Puerto Rico upon completion of the requisite licensing requirements. All Ross students who are U.S. citizens/permanent residents and meet the Department of Education criteria are eligible for Federal Stafford Loans and Federal Graduate PLUS Loans.

Application Information

For specific application information (availability, deadlines, fees, VMCAS participation, and supplemental application requirements), please refer to the contact information listed above.

Evaluation Criteria:

Scholastic record, including cumulative grade point average (GPA) in prerequisite courses

Competitive Graduate Record Examination (GRE) scores

Application essay

Pre-veterinary committee evaluations

Letters of recommendation from academic and/or professional references

Extracurricular activities and accomplishments

Personal qualities

Record of experience working with animals

Personal interview

Prerequisites for Admission

Course Requirements and semester hours:

General Biology with laboratory	2 semesters or 8 credit hours
General Chemistry with laboratory	2 semesters or 8 credit hours
Organic Chemistry with laboratory	1 semester or 4 credit hours
Physics with laboratory	1 semester or 4 credit hours
Biochemistry	1 semester or 3 credit hours
Upper Level Biology	3 semesters or 12 credit hours
English*	2 semesters or 8 credit hours
Mathematics	1 semester or 3 credit hours

* *Canadian students may satisfy the English requirement using year 13 English or Composition.*

Course completion deadline: Required courses must be completed prior to enrollment.

AP credit policy: Must appear on official college transcripts.

Standardized Examinations: Results of the Graduate Record Examination (GRE) are required. Applicants presenting fewer than 60 upper division credits from a college or university must provide the official record of the scores for the Test of English as a Foreign Language (TOEFL). The minimum acceptable score is 550 on the paper-based test, or 213 on the computer-based test.

Additional requirements and considerations: It is highly desirable that applicants complete the equivalent of at least six weeks of full-time practical experience, working with large domesticated animals (e.g., cows, horses, sheep, goats, pigs) and small domestic animals (e.g., dogs, cats). It is preferable that all such experience has taken place under the supervision of a practicing veterinarian, but comparable experience may be considered.

Summary of Admission Procedure

Timetable

> Application deadline: None; rolling admissions
> Date interviews are held: Year-round
> Date acceptances mailed: As soon as possible after the interview
> School begins: Three start dates per year: September, January and May

Deposit (to hold place in class): $1,000.00

Deferments: Considered

2008–2009 admissions summary

	Number of Applicants	Number of New Entrants
Nonresident	1,013	325

Expenses for the 2009–2010 Academic Year (subject to change)

Tuition and fees

Nonresident	$38,695

Dual-Degree Program

Ross University School of Veterinary Medicine has dual degree agreements with several undergraduate institutions. Under this program, any undergraduate junior who meets the set standards will be accepted the following year at Ross University School of Veterinary Medicine, and the undergraduate institution agrees to grant its baccalaureate degree to students who successfully complete the first two academic semesters at Ross University. The undergraduate institution will have the sole discretion to determine the field of study in which the baccalaureate degree is awarded.

St. George's University

Office of Admission
St. George's University
c/o The North American Correspondent
University Support Services, LLC
One East Main Street
Bay Shore, NY 11706-8399
Phone +1 (631) 665-8500
US/Canada Toll-Free 1(800) 899-6337
UK Free Phone: 0800 1699061
Fax: +1 (631) 665-5590
E-mail: sguinfo@sgu.edu
Website: www.sgu.edu

St. George's University School of Veterinary Medicine is proud to be in its eleventh year of academic excellence exemplified by its breadth of highly regarded education, unprecedented student support services, and internationally recognized faculty. The core mission of the University is creating excellent academic programs within an international setting where students and faculty are actively recruited from around the world. St. George's University has drawn faculty and students from over 140 countries, assembling a diverse community of disparate cultural and educational backgrounds.

Located on the southwest corner of the Caribbean island of Grenada, SGU's shoreline location offers its growing student body a serene environment in which to live, learn and create a worldwide network of friends and colleagues. Along with SGU's state-of-the-art facilities, complete with a large animal farm, marine station, and the SGU Small Animal Hospital, St. George's University School of Veterinary Medicine prepares its students for leadership, life-long success and service in a constantly changing world.

Over 5,000 students from throughout the world are enrolled in one of the three University's Schools: Medicine, Veterinary Medicine, and Arts and Sciences. SGU students also benefit from world-renowned international academic partnerships with universities, hospitals and other educational and scientific institutions.

The veterinary medical program is delivered with a number of entry options: the seven-, six- and five-year programs which begin with the preveterinary medical sciences and an option to enter directly into the four-year veterinary medical program. This enables students flexible entry points depending upon their academic backgrounds. Students accepted into the preveterinary medical sciences are placed in the appropriate program option (either the seven-, six-

or five-year program track) according to their academic background and are enrolled in the veterinary medical program for five to seven years. Applicants accepted directly into the veterinary medical sciences generally complete the program in four years.

The DVM program is conducted on the University's main campus on the True Blue peninsula of Grenada, West Indies, except for the final year which is the clinical year spent at an affiliated AVMA-accredited School of Veterinary Medicine. These schools are located in the United States, Canada, United Kingdom, Ireland, and Australia.

Prerequisites for Admission

The requirements for direct entry into the four-year DVM program vary depending on the educational system of your home country. What is required for all applicants is completion of secondary school, a period of farm experience or time spent in a veterinary practice, and possession of a bachelor's degree from an accredited University or 90 credit hours.

The following specific undergraduate coursework (or its equivalent) is required as part of the preveterinary medical sciences requirements for admission (credit hours):

   One year: General Biology or Zoology with lab (8)
   One year: Inorganic Chemistry (General or Physical) with lab (8)
   One semester: Organic Chemistry with lab (4)
   One semester: Biochemistry (3)
   One semester: Genetics (3)
   One semester: Physics with lab (4)
   One semester: Calculus, Computer Science or Statistics (3)
   One semester: English (3)

Applicants from North America

A completed bachelor's degree from an accredited university is required for direct entry into the four-year veterinary medical program. A candidate may apply before completion of the bachelor's degree; however, a candidate's acceptance will be withdrawn if the degree is not obtained.

Standardized Examination: Candidates must submit scores on the Graduate Record Examination or alternatively on the MCAT. (Our GRE Code is 7153; MCAT code 21303.)

A minimum of two letters of recommendation, (preferably from science professors) or a preveterinary medical committee evaluation, are required.

Applicants from the British System of Education

For direct entry into the four-year DVM program, a bachelor's degree with a strong science background is required.

Applicants with passes at the Advanced Level of the General Certificate of Education will be assessed individually and will be considered for appropriate entry into the five-year DVM program. Generally A Level students with the appropriate courses and grades matriculate into the five-year veterinary medical program.

If English is not the principal language, the applicant must have achieved a score in the Test of English as a Foreign Language (TOEFL) of at least 600 points (written) or 250 points (computer-based).

Applicants from Other Systems of Education

An applicant must have achieved the successful completion of secondary school (twelve years post-kindergarten, comprising four years post-primary/elementary, that, in itself is at least eight years long), preferably in a science curriculum or track.

An applicant must have completed a bachelor's degree (or its equivalent), which includes a science background and the study of English.

If English is not the principal language, the applicant must have achieved a score in the Test of English as a Foreign Language (TOEFL) of at least 600 points (written) or 250 points (computer-based).

Applicants who do not meet the admission requirements for direct entry into the four-year DVM program may apply for admission to either the seven-, six-, or five-year veterinary medical program that begin with the preveterinary medical sciences. Depending on the country of origin and academic background, a student enters the preveterinary medical sciences for a period of one to three years, with the full veterinary program ranging from four to seven years, depending upon the individual's point of entry.

Application Deadlines for August and January Matriculation

The School of Veterinary Medicine begins first-term classes in mid-August and again in mid-January. The Committee on Admission utilizes a rolling admission policy in the School of Veterinary Medicine; therefore applications are accepted and reviewed on an ongoing basis. The final deadline for receipt of applications and all supporting documentation is June 15th of the current year for the August class and November 15th of the preceding year for the January class.

Prospective candidates should note that entering classes are highly competitive and applications completed early have the advantage of being reviewed at the beginning of the admission's process.

The time necessary to secure official transcripts, standardized test scores and letters of recommendation should be taken into consideration. The Committee reserves the right to defer an application to the following semester if there are no available seats.

Interview:

The Office of Admission encourages candidates who have been approved for an interview to request interviews in Grenada and will schedule one upon the applicant's request. The University recognizes that financial considerations may prevent many candidates who reside at great distances from Grenada from choosing this option. Interviews, therefore, may be conducted in the United States, the United Kingdom, Africa, the Middle East, the Far East, the Caribbean or other locations that best serve the diverse applicant pool. Interviews are conducted by faculty members, visiting professors, or graduates of St. George's University and are mandatory for acceptance into the veterinary medical program.

Candidates are advised that being granted an interview is no guarantee of acceptance; the interview itself plays a significant part in the decision by the Committee on Admission.

2009 admissions summary

January 2009 incoming class:

Total Applicants:	122	Entering Students:	46
US Applicants	108	US Applicants	40
Non US	14	Non US	06

August 2009 incoming class:

Total Applicants:	252	Entering Students:	76
US Applicants	227	US Applicants	71
Non US	25	Non US	05

Expenses for 2009 incoming students

Tuition and Fees are the same for all DVM students regardless of residence:

Years 1-3 (non-clinical years in Grenada) $26,256 yearly

Year   4   (clinical year at affiliated university) $45,720

Dual Degree Programs:

Combined DVM / MPH, MSc, and MBA degree programs are available.

Applications can be submitted online directly through the SGU website at www.sgu.edu, or via a hard copy which can be obtained by speaking with one of our enrolment counselors at 1 (800) 899-6337 ext 280.

St. Matthew's University

School of Veterinary Medicine
Campus:
P.O. Box 32330
Grand Cayman KY1-1209
CAYMAN ISLANDS
Telephone: 345-745-3199

Administrative Office:
12124 High Tech Ave., Suite 350
Orlando, FL 32817
Telephone: 800.498.9700
Email: admissions@stmatthews.edu
www.stmatthews.edu

St. Matthew's University School of Veterinary Medicine is located on beautiful Grand Cayman in the Caribbean. Grand Cayman is the fifth largest financial district in the world and has a highly developed infrastructure comparable to the United States. It is also one of the safest islands in the Caribbean boasting one of the lowest crime and poverty rates.

The School of Veterinary Medicine offers students a veterinary medical education program focused on patient-centered care as the foundation of the program.

The School has facilities at the main campus close to Seven Mile Beach plus a new Clinical Teaching Facility located in the middle of the island where it is closer to the main livestock populations. In addition to surgery, medicine and clinical skills instruction at this facility, anatomy and pathology laboratories are also held there. Transportation is available from the main campus to the Teaching Facility. Students have the opportunity to travel to local farms with veterinary staff from the Cayman Department of Agriculture. Presently the students spend seven (7) semesters on Grand Cayman and their final 12 months in clinical programs at one of our seven Clinical Program Affiliate Schools in the US.

There are significant opportunities for students to gain experience with exotic species through our collaborations with the Cayman Turtle Farm, Central Caribbean Marine Institute, Dolphin Discovery, the Blue Iguana Project and the Coral Reef Research Program.

Application Information

For specific application information (availability, deadlines, fees, transferring to SMU, and VMCAS participation), please refer to the contact information listed above.

Prerequisites for Admission

Course Requirements and semester hours:

General Biology*	8
General Chemistry*	8
Organic Chemistry*	4
Biochemistry	3
Language Arts (English)	6
College Math or Computer Science	3
Physics (Recommended)	4
Social Science (Recommended)	6

These courses must include an attached laboratory.

Course completion deadline: all prerequisite courses must be completed prior to matriculation.

Standardized Examinations: Graduate Record Examination (GRE®), general test, is not required but strongly recommended. The exam must have been taken within the previous 5 calendar years, and scores must be sent to the Office of Admissions as part of the application for admission.

Additional Considerations: Each candidate is carefully evaluated on the basis of these factors:

Academic background
Overall grade point average
Science grade point average
Strength of major/minor
GRE scores
Letters of reference
Personal statement
College activities that demonstrate service to the community
Personal Interview (by invitation)

Summary of Admission Procedure

Timetable

Application deadlines: None. Rolling admissions. Three semester starts.
Interviews: Held in person or via telephone.
Acceptance notification: Within 7-10 business days.
School begins: August, January, May

Deposit (to hold place in class): $500.00

Deferments: Considered on an individual basis. A non-refundable fee ($500) is assessed if deferment is approved.

Evaluation criteria: The 3-part admission procedure includes an objective evaluation of academic credentials, a subjective review of personal credentials, and an interview by invitation.

Transfer: transfer credits (advanced standing) may be awarded at the discretion of the University.

Expenses for the 2009–2010 Academic Year

Tuition and fees
Basic Sciences	$9,375
Clinical Sciences	$15,525
Additional fees	$275

Dual-Degree Programs

MBA graduate degree program is available.
Visit our site at http://www.stmatthews.edu/vet_curriculum_concurrent-degree-program.shtml

POLICIES ON ADVANCED STANDING

Transfers are permitted to most colleges of veterinary medicine in the United States under specified conditions. Typical requirements include a vacancy in the class, completion of all prerequisite requirements, and compatible curricula. Following is a listing of schools and some of the conditions under which they will consider a transfer from another veterinary college with advanced standing. More detailed information may be obtained by writing to the individual schools in which you have an interest.

UNITED STATES

University of Florida
1. An opening must exist in the second- or third-year class.
2. Students are only rarely considered for advanced standing based on exceptional personal circumstances.
3. Student must be enrolled in an AVMA accredited college.
4. Student must meet all prerequisites for admission as a first-year student (including GRE® scores).
5. The curricula of the two schools must be sufficiently alike to allow a student to enter without deficiencies in academic background.
6. Applicant must not have been denied admission to the University of Florida College of Veterinary Medicine as a first-year student.
7. Applicants must have a letter approving transfer from their dean or associate dean.

University of Georgia
1. Priority is given to Georgia residents, followed by contract state residents, then all other applicants.
2. Applicants will be considered for entry in the second or third year.
3. Applications must include a letter of support written by a senior administrator of the school in which the applicant is currently enrolled.
4. All selection criteria for regular applicants apply to transfer applicants.
5. No individual is eligible for transfer who has been dismissed or is on probation at any other school or college for deficiency in scholarship or because of misconduct.

University of Illinois

1. Transfer students will only be considered for the beginning of the second year of veterinary medicine and only if transfer seats become available in that class.
2. All prerequisite science courses must be completed prior to the request for transfer.
3. Minimum grade requirements include:
    cumulative and science GPAs of 2.75 on a 4.00 scale (doesn't include veterinary work);
    results of the Graduate Record Examination General Test completed within the last two years.
4. Student must complete the same preveterinary coursework as required for students accepted to the first year of the program.
5. Student must be in good academic standing.
6. To be considered for transfer, a student must present credentials for *preprofessional work* that fulfill the University of Illinois College of Veterinary Medicine requirements for first-year entry.
7. Complete information and an application can be found at vetmed.illinois.edu/asa/brochure.

Cornell University

Cornell University does not accept transfer credit.

Iowa State University

Acceptance of students for advanced standing is on the recommendation of the Academic Standards Committee. Space must be available in the class to which the student is applying. See website, http://vetmed.iastate.edu/academics/prospective-students/admissions/transfer-admissions, for the transfer application form and further details.

Kansas State University

Acceptance of students for advanced standing is on recommendation of the Admissions Committee on a space-available basis.

Louisiana State University

1. There must be a vacancy in the class.
2. The curricula must be compatible.
3. The student must be in good academic standing with at least a 3.2 GPA in veterinary coursework at his/her present college.
4. Admission is limited to the second year of the program and only into the fall semester.

5. Each request for transfer is considered on a case-by-case basis.
6. To initiate the transfer process, please carefully read the DVM Transfer Guidelines information at www.vetmed.lsu.edu/admissions/transfer_apps.asp.

Michigan State University

1. Admission consideration is offered only to those current matriculants in professional veterinary curricula who believe that there are extenuating circumstances that would precipitate significant undue hardship if they continue at their current institution.
2. Applicants must also demonstrate quality academic performance throughout their professional school enrollment.
3. The curricula of the two schools must be sufficiently alike to allow a student to enter the second-year class without deficiencies in academic background.
4. All selection criteria for regular applicants apply to transfer applicants.
5. Priority is given to Michigan residents.
6. Space must be available.
7. AVMA accreditation of current school is considered.

University of Minnesota

1. Transfers are not allowed to any specific requested year or semester. The committee will place each applicant in the year or semester of the curriculum deemed appropriate after analysis of equivalency of the required courses involved.
2. No academic work or standing will be accepted from DVM curricula other than those deemed accredited ("AVMA accredited") by the American Veterinary Medical Association.
3. All applicants must be U.S. citizens, be holders of permanent resident alien visas, or have achieved landed immigrant status.
4. All applicants are required to have finished at least one full academic year at the institution from which transfer is requested and must be in good academic standing at the time of discontinuance according to written verification from the institution.
5. All applicants must document that not more than two calendar years have elapsed between discontinuance and application to our DVM program.
6. All applicants must have achieved a cumulative GPA of 3.00 (of 4.00) for the required courses at the initial institution.
7. Please visit the following website for more details: http://www.cvm.umn.edu/education/prospective/TransferStudents/home.html

Mississippi State University

Transfer students are accepted on a limited basis to fill vacancies in the freshman or sophomore class.

1. Any applicant must be in good academic standing, never have failed a course while in veterinary medical school, and never have been dismissed from a veterinary school.
2. Applicants considered for transfer admission will be required to attend an interview at Mississippi State University.
3. No transfer applicant is accepted at a point later than the first semester of the sophomore year. All veterinary medical students must complete at least three years at Mississippi State University to be eligible for a degree.
4. Students accepted into the phase 1 freshman or sophomore year are required to meet the College's current computer requirements.

For more information, contact Kim Higgason, Administrative Assistant, 663-325-4161, higgason@cvm.msstate.edu.

University of Missouri

1. Must be a vacancy in the class.
2. Will consider students who are U.S. citizens or holders of permanent alien visas and who have finished at least two years in a college of veterinary medicine that is AVMA accredited.
3. Students must be in good academic standing, and a letter of reference from the dean's office of the present college is required.

North Carolina State University

1. Must be a vacancy in the class.
2. Consideration by the Admission Committee on an individual basis.
3. Curricula must be compatible.
4. A letter from the dean of the current school certifying the applicant's academic standing.
5. Letter of recommendation from a faculty member at the original college.
6. Only accept transfers from AVMA accredited colleges.
7. At least 50% of DVM credit hours should be completed at North Carolina State in order to earn a North Carolina State University degree.

Ohio State University

1. An opening must exist.
2. Student must be enrolled in an AVMA accredited college.
3. The curricula of the two schools must be sufficiently alike to allow the student to enter a class without deficiencies in his or her academic background.

4. Student must be in good academic standing in his or her present college and have a supporting letter from the Dean of Student and Academic Affairs to this effect.
5. Each request for transfer is considered on an individual basis, taking into account personal hardship, family situations, etc.
6. Must meet same prerequisite requirements as first-year applicants.

Oklahoma State University

Transfer students are considered. Each application is evaluated on an individual basis. See website for transfer guide. http://www.cvhs.okstate.edu/files/Future%20Students/TransferApp.pdf

Oregon State University

Admission of students with advanced standing is considered only in certain circumstances, and each case is considered on an individual basis.

University of Pennsylvania

PennVet does not consider transfer applications.

Purdue University

1. Positions must be available in the relevant class.
2. Student must have legitimate ties to the State of Indiana or extenuating/personal circumstance (e.g., transfer of spouse to Indiana for employment purposes).
3. Student must be in good academic standing in his/her present program.
4. Students must have completed 1–2 years of DVM courses with an **exceptional** academic record in those courses.
5. Veterinary medical curricula must be compatible.
6. Student must have support of the administration from the program in which he/she is currently enrolled.

University of Tennessee

Admission of students with advanced standing may be considered for unique circumstances on a case-by-case basis. Space must be available in the class and the professional curricula must reasonably match between the schools. The Admissions Committee will review applicants' credentials and interview those determined to best meet admission criteria. Admission is usually limited to the second semester of the first year of the professional curriculum. Students must be in good standing at their present college.

Texas A & M University

Students requesting advanced standing must meet the following requirements:

1. Must have completed all previous professional veterinary courses in an AVMA accredited college of veterinary medicine.
2. Must have successfully completed the academic term preceding the semester into which student requests admission.
3. Must comply with all requirements for transfer into the university as described in the current catalog.
4. May request transfer only into the second through seventh semesters of the professional curriculum.
5. At the time of matriculation the student must certify by letter that he/she has not been convicted of crimes in the period from first enrollment in the college of veterinary medicine from which the student desires transfer until date of matriculation at Texas A&M University.
6. To request transfer consideration, the student must meet all requirements as posted on the College website at http://www.cvm.tamu.edu/dcvm/admissions/transferpol.shtml.

Tufts University

Applicants from other veterinary schools are considered. Students with advanced standing are admitted if and when space becomes available in the second-year class. The application deadline is June 1 for the following September.

Tuskegee University

TUSVM does not accept transfer applications.

Washington State University

Admission of students with advanced standing is considered only in very specific and unique circumstances, and each case is considered on an individual basis.

University of Wisconsin

Wisconsin does not accept advanced standing students for admission.

INTERNATIONAL

Massey University

Applications for admission with advanced standing will only be considered by students enrolled in a veterinary program with a compatible curriculum, and pending an available space in the appropriate stage of the program. Applicants should contact Vetschool@massey.ac.nz to apply for advanced standing. Applicants are advised that vacancies are uncommon.

Murdoch University

Applications for advanced standing will only be considered from students whose studies have been completed in a DVM program. Applicants are required to apply formally for advanced standing and provide the necessary documentation to allow for a full comparison between the previous study and Murdoch University's unit requirements. Prior courses must duplicate or substantially overlap multiple factors including breadth and depth of content, duration, objectives, assessment, context, and academic standard (level of intellectual effort required) for exemption to be granted.

University of Calgary

Applications for admission to advanced semesters may be considered from students who have been enrolled in DVM programs at other institutions, subject to the availability of spaces in the DVM Program and the academic standing of the candidate. When places are available, candidates may be asked to present themselves for an interview and may be asked to pass examinations on subject matter in the veterinary curriculum. Applicants are advised that vacancies are rare and that restrictions on residency and citizenship status may be applied.

University of Guelph

Applications for admission to advanced semesters will be considered from students who have been enrolled in DVM programs at other institutions, subject to the availability of spaces in the DVM Program and the academic standing of the candidate. When places are available, candidates may be asked to present themselves for an interview and may be asked to pass examinations on subject matter in the veterinary curriculum. Applicants are advised that vacancies are rare.

University of Prince Edward Island

Applicants who have completed all or portions of a veterinary medical program may apply for advanced standing to the second year of the DVM program.

Applicants for advanced standing must present evidence of educational accomplishments and may be required to address missing courses or competencies expected of our incoming second-year students. Students admitted with advanced standing must begin the college year in September.

The candidate must file a formal application and may be interviewed by the Admissions Committee and possibly other faculty. Places for admission to the college with advanced standing are limited and depend on vacancies.

It is imperative that the Admissions Committee have detailed and translated summaries of veterinary medical academic programs and accomplishments for those seeking advanced placement from schools in foreign countries.

Advanced-standing applications should be on file and completed as early as possible and no later than January 1. Candidates are strongly encouraged to visit the website http://www.upei.ca/registrar/3_prof_degree_dvm.

University of Saskatchewan

Applications for admission with advanced standing will only be considered if a vacancy in the Year II class develops. Students applying for advanced standing must meet the normal residency requirements and must be enrolled in a program that has a compatible curriculum. Applicants are required to complete a formal application form and, dependant on their academic record, will be considered for an interview. Part of the interview will be an assessment of their current knowledge. Applicants will be required to submit a recent GRE score and, if English is not their first language, will also be required to submit a TOEFL score. Admission is not considered beyond the second year of the program.

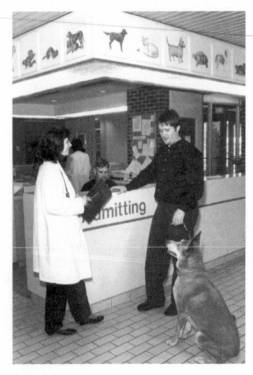

Small-animal care in a clinic is but one of many options for hands-on training at veterinary medical colleges. Photo courtesy of Atlantic Veterinary College, University of Prince Edward Island.

APPLICATION AND ENROLLMENT DATA

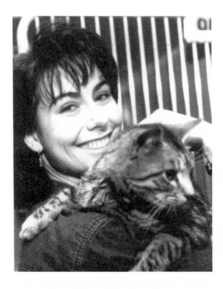

Job satisfaction: giving a little TLC during clinical rounds. Photo by Vivian Dixon, courtesy of University of Georgia College of Veterinary Medicine.

Table 1

Applicants to U.S. Colleges of Veterinary Medicine
by Residence, 2003–2010

VMCAS Data Only

State	2003	2004	2005	2006	2007	2008	2009	2010
Alberta	3	2	5	1	5	6	3	
Alaska	8	7	7	6	3	4	9	8
Alabama	23	28	15	106	108	117	105	92
Arkansas	31	38	41	31	40	40	35	36
Arizona	75	92	78	81	76	94	85	92
British	4	6	6	3	2	7	7	5
California	335	329	367	557	589	651	655	611
Colorado	295	245	247	247	228	224	253	277
Connecticut	39	36	37	36	58	60	56	60
Washington, DC	5	3	4	5	6	7	6	5
Delaware	10	15	15	10	15	11	16	10
Florida	255	264	271	292	324	332	326	311
Foreign	18	18	22	16	26	13	43	43
Georgia	215	170	192	174	194	190	194	189
Guam	1	1	0	0	1	0	0	0
Hawaii	17	23	17	11	20	25	34	30
Iowa	11	16	17	112	120	116	118	139
Idaho	12	21	16	23	15	24	40	23
Illinois	216	212	227	232	223	231	249	253
Indiana	102	115	110	112	122	107	120	121
Kansas	17	17	19	20	134	132	130	144
Kentucky	33	39	41	124	106	101	91	103
Louisiana	152	142	132	124	137	150	148	129
Massachusetts	95	97	96	106	121	127	119	106
Manitoba	3	0	1	3	4	3	8	4
Maryland	105	102	79	106	118	114	130	109
Maine	11	14	16	18	16	17	18	31
Michigan	214	226	208	241	243	246	241	220
Minnesota	141	158	159	177	174	186	182	189
Missouri	20	22	21	20	25	34	31	35
Mississippi	64	58	56	56	52	54	70	64

Table 1 (continued)

State	2003	2004	2005	2006	2007	2008	2009	2010
Montana	27	28	20	28	33	24	30	26
North Carolina	201	175	197	224	205	193	225	214
North Dakota	21	14	20	23	21	24	23	27
Nebraska	12	23	26	47	53	49	54	69
New Brunswick	0	0	0	0	0	0	1	0
New Hampshire	16	19	24	16	20	22	21	25
New Jersey	109	116	103	107	133	135	115	109
New Mexico	27	47	38	24	32	38	36	35
Nova Scotia	0	1	2	0	1	0	1	2
Nevada	23	23	24	26	21	22	25	24
New York	209	197	262	282	269	265	263	248
Ohio	90	123	79	102	304	264	273	304
Oklahoma	8	11	7	18	20	132	116	122
Ontario	5	9	10	16	16	22	25	20
Oregon	84	87	76	98	94	103	99	79
Pennsylvania	230	259	232	243	266	265	267	262
Prince Edward Island	0	0	0	0	1	0	0	1
Province of Quebec	0	0	0	0	0	1	3	3
Puerto Rico	32	36	24	34	29	27	29	41
Rhode Island	10	10	9	9	7	12	17	18
South Carolina	75	67	57	66	65	64	85	68
South Dakota	18	8	16	14	11	17	18	23
Saskatchewan	0	0	0	1	0	0	4	1
Tennessee	121	101	132	138	134	149	169	153
U.S. Territories	1	0	1	1	1	0	0	0
Texas	101	139	139	132	187	149	189	213
Utah	29	33	33	32	31	32	26	31
Virginia	162	151	159	186	193	190	193	176
Virgin Islands	0	1	0	1	0	0	0	2
Vermont	10	10	11	8	13	17	11	16
Washington	61	58	51	48	68	79	148	132
Wisconsin	159	135	154	164	158	153	175	196
West Virginia	36	24	34	36	29	27	32	41
Wyoming	23	19	21	20	20	22	13	15

Table 2

Applicant Data for Classes 2003–2010

Applications by College

VMCAS Data Only

College 2003 2004	2003	2004	2005	2006	2007	2008	2009	2010
Auburn University	555	585	638	869**	860	824	759	667
Colorado State University	1,447	1,402	1,475	1,482	1,639	1,701	1,877	1,773
Cornell University	437	464**	872	853	888	910	902	868
Iowa State University	464	510	553	647**	819	968	1,043	1,057
Kansas State University	315	425	498	603	998**	1,102	1,231	1,202
Louisiana State University	818	774	799	658	698	712	638	667
Massey University	*	*	*	*	144	166	152	126
Michigan State University	1,010	1,015	884	1,008	761	861	943	902
Mississippi State University	378	636	381	369	400	479	760	813
Murdoch International	*	*	*	*	*	*	86	85
North Carolina State University	518	513	564	600	493	482	553	725
Ohio State University	579	579	553	544	1,000**	874	794	792
Oklahoma State University	237	252	286	278	351	436**	452	467
Oregon State University	661	668	630	663	759	554	509	455
Purdue University	630	611	590	583	749	785	698	674
Royal Veterinary College	*	*	*	*	*	291	271	275

Table 2 (continued)

University College Dublin	*	*	*	*	*	*	95	170
University of California, Davis	393	413	402	966**	1,120	1,178	1,135	1,057
University of Edinburgh	*	101	132	169	224	255	195	215
University of Florida	697	752	770	799	896	897	871	822
University of Georgia	607	547	566	524	543	495	567	551
University of Glasgow	225	193	172	181	216	262	224	205
University of Guelph-Ontario Veterinary College	43	80	104	96	113	132	85	133
University of Illinois	758	741	753	809	921	842	860	781
University of Minnesota	643	655	751	916	1,010	1,153	1,083	1,025
University of Missouri	143	138	83	428	609	618	698	765
University of PEI-Atlantic Veterinary College	213	190	186	187	212	280	262	217
University of Pennsylvania	1,110	1,216	1,246	1,291	1,475	1,466	1,359	1,209
University of Tennessee	269	464	768	763	760	757	824	851
University of Wisconsin	830	792	868	987	1,144	887	1,134	1,046
Virginia-Maryland Regional College	761	745	785	872	914	838	892	858
Washington State University	562	617	647	641	830	892	865	929
Western University of Health Sciences	*	326	375	557	605	775**	754	754

* Was not a member of VMCAS in the year indicated.

** Indicates the year the college shifted from limited participation to full participation with VMCAS

Table 3

Applicant Data for Classes 2003 - 2010

Age Distribution

VMCAS Data Only

Age	2003	2004	2005	2006	2007	2008	2009	2010
20	396	408	357	412	465	457	519	486
21	1,132	1,179	1,258	1,374	1,573	1,619	1,655	1,729
22	777	773	890	980	1,069	1,105	1,116	1,171
23	523	534	563	680	713	746	748	722
24	368	323	349	365	506	490	490	524
25-30	861	831	802	998	1,033	1,092	1,123	1,096
31-35	199	214	197	181	192	210	176	160
Other	193	191	165	204	189	201	381	255
	2003	2004	2005	2006	2007	2008	2009	2010
Number of Applicants	4,449	4,453	4,581	5,194	5,740	5,920	6,208	6,143

Table 4
Applicant Data for Classes 2003 - 2010
Gender Distribution
VMCAS Data Only

	2003 (% of pool)	2004 (% of pool)	2005 (% of pool)	2006 (% of pool)
Number of Applicants	4,449	4,453	4,581	5,194
Applicant who identified gender	4,445	4,450	4,579	5,192
Total # of Females who identified gender	3,545 (79.68)	3,518 (79)	3,682 (80.38)	4,147 (79.84)
Total # of Males who identified gender	900 (20.23)	932 (20.93)	897 (19.59)	1,045 (20.12)
Other				
% Change from:		*2003/2004*	*2004/2005*	*2005/2006*
Female		-0.76%	4.66%	12.63%
Male		3.56%	-3.76%	16.49%

207

Table 4 (continued)

2007 (% of pool)	2008 (% of pool)	2009 (% of pool)	2010 (% of pool)
5,740	5,920	6,208	6,143
5,738	5,913	5,972	5,895
4,562 (79.48)	4,703 (79.44)	4,715 (78.95)	4,683 (79.44)
1,176 (20.49)	1,210 (20.44)	1,257 (21.04)	1,212 (20.56)

2006/2007	2007/2008	2008/2009	2009/2010
10.00%	3.09%	.026%	0.68%
12.54%	2.89%	3.88%	-3.58%

Table 5

Applicant Data for Classes 2003–20010

	2003	(% response)
Number of Applicants	4449	
Number of applicants who responded to at least one race	4107	92.31%
Number of applicants who responded to two or more race	96	2.16%

Ethnicity:

Hispanic - Yes	++	++
Hispanic - No	++	++

Race:

African-American / Black	75	1.69%
Spanish / Hispanic / Latino American	*	*
No Spanish / Hispanic / Latino American	*	*
Hispanic American	107	2.41%
Mexican / Mexican American / Chicano	40	0.89%
Puerto Rican	**	**
Cuban	**	**
Other Spanish / Hispanic / Latino American	**	**
Other Latino / Spanish American	66	1.48%
American Indian / Alaskan Native	41	0.92%
Filipino / Filipino American (Counted as Asian)	17	0.38%
Chinese / Chinese American (Counted as Asian)	49	1.10%
Japanese / Japanese American (Counted as Asian)	30	0.67%
Korean / Korean American (Counted as Asian)	25	0.56%
Pacific Islander	10	0.23%
Asian	21	0.47%
Caucasian / Middle Eastern	3684	82.81%
Other	47	1.06%

Special Note: For the years 2003–2005 VMCAS has always categorized Spanish/Hispanic/Latino as a race.

Table 5 (continued)

2004	(% response)	2005	(% response)	2006	(% response)	2007	(% response)
4453		4581		5194		5740	
4043	91.02%	4214	91.99%	4551	87.62%	5002	87.14%
103	2.31%	115	2.15%	3040	58.52%	3403	59.29%
++	++	++	++	++	++	++	++
++	++	++	++	++	++	++	++
72	1.62%	87	1.89%	82	1.58%	110	1.92%
*	*	*		306	5.89%	293	5.10%
*	*	*		2762	53.18%	3139	54.69%
106	2.38%	128	2.79%	***	***	***	***
44	0.98%	51	1.11%	94	1.81%	94	1.64%
**	**	**		72	1.39%	57	0.99%
**	**	**		30	0.58%	29	0.51%
**	**	**		112	2.16%	116	2.02%
56	1.26%	65	1.42%	***	***	***	***
44	0.98%	53	1.16%	63	1.21%	60	1.05%
13	0.29%	15	0.33%	26	0.50%	28	0.49%
74	1.66%	70	1.53%	74	1.42%	91	1.59%
48	1.08%	42	0.92%	52	1.00%	61	1.06%
30	0.67%	23	0.50%	38	0.73%	42	0.73%
12	0.27%	8	0.18%	8	0.15%	21	0.37%
22	0.49%	23	0.50%	37	0.71%	41	0.71%
3574	80.26%	3710	80.99%	3966	76.36%	4358	75.92%
51	1.15%	57	1.24%	64	1.23%	83	1.45%

Beginning with the VMCAS 2010 cycle, VMCAS has aligned with standard census reporting. As such, there are a number of categories that have been retired (+) and folded into other categories.

Table 5 (continued)

2008	(% response)	2009	(% response)	2010	(% response)
5920		6208		6143	
5149	86.98%	5778	93.07%	4787	77.93%
3507	59.24%	3317	53.43%	1356	22.07%
++	++	++	++	374	6.09%
++	++	++	++	5225	85.06%
121	2.04%	135	2.17%	113	1.84%
326	5.51%	335	5.40%	***	***
3209	54.21%	4539	73.12%	***	***
***	***	***	***	***	***
102	1.72%	99	1.59%	***	***
68	1.15%	72	1.16%	***	***
37	0.63%	30	0.48%	***	***
103	1.74%	122	1.97%	***	***
***	***	***	***	***	***
114	1.93%	82	1.32%	115	1.87%
25	0.42%	31	0.50%	+	+
101	1.71%	108	1.74%	+	+
57	0.96%	64	1.03%	+	+
56	0.95%	65	1.05%	+	+
16	0.27%	12	0.19%	25	0.41%
57	0.96%	62	1.00%	315	5.13%
4437	74.95%	4743	76.40%	4319	70.31%
77	1.30%	96	1.55%	-	-

* in 2006 this category choice was moved to the heading of Ethnicity; ** was added as a specific ethnicity identifier; *** re-categorized under ethnicity; ++ Not reported prior to 2010.

VMCAS fills between 59–75% of the seats to Vet Colleges; VMCAS is seen as representative of the entire pool of applicants.

Table 6

Sources of Financial Aid for 2008-2009 Academic Year

TITLE IV

School	Perkins (NDSL) Loan		(Total) Stafford Loan		Un-Subsidized Stafford		Pell Grants	
	Amount	No.	Amount	No.	Amount	No.	Amount	No.
AUB	2,000	1	2,500,065	80	5,615,131	77		
UCD	545,972	144	3,380,519	408	9,336,957	375		
CSU			3,652,697	439	7,812,088	395		
COR	386,950	190	2,405,978	286	5,345,444	260		
FLA			2,253,678	295	6,474,146	297		
UGA	14,000	7	8,489,158	299	6,038,136	275	116,626	7
ILL			3,148,200	382	8,998,366	355		
ISU			12,925,559	438	8,230,085	396		
KSU	199,200	119	11,450,038	372	8,362,344	332	1,723,243	129
LSU	90,000	15	2,164,090	258	5,250,485	229		
MSU			3,922,850	388	3,912,983	387		
MIN	24,000	4	3,124,114	80	8,141,942	79		
MIS			2,156,872	255	6,088,049	237		
UMO	97,000	76	2,357,955	280	5,420,589	246		

Table 6 (continued)

NCSU			2,065,853	247	3,893,711	219	5,412,700	
OSU			4,193,506	501	4,959,485	238		469
OKL	1,100	1	2,146,360	258	3,227,609	42		
ORE	147,108	34	1,537,315	43				
PENN	313,880	107	15,130,854	381	12,002,854	381		
PUR			1,767,367	225	3,483,539	191		
TENN	174,640	48	5,679,515	263	13,725,483	252		
TAMU	581,288	268	6,333,168	477	5,178,974	477		
TUF	174,000	29	1,989,979	239	6,088,595	225		
TUS			401,210	39	456,280	41		
VMR	344,866	59	8,940,764	303	6,191,708	271		
WSU	2,000	2	2,792,175	341	6,255,592	322	22,145	6
WES			2,825,896	335	10,943,751	328		
WIS	333,000	111	2,320,425	277	5,698,540	271		
CLG								
ONT								
MON	990,935	306						
PEI			1,484,500	73	864,000	72		
SKW								

"No." indicates the number of students

Table 6 *(continued)*

| | TITLE VII | | | | | | | | OTHER | |
| HPSL | | HEAL | | LDS | | SDS | | Other Loans | |
Amount	No.	Amount	No.	Amount	No.	Amount	No.	Amount	No.
117,000	15							167,014	10
208,967	63							55,190	13
224,000	112			12,000	3			87,512	9
189,510	42					87,110	19	62,925	7
72,000	6								
504,000	91	211,900	72	59,500	35	190,554	63	2,648,198	224
581,271	132							639,137	67
299,115	48			10,000	6			732,134	46
542,500	44							641,578	51
389,000	87							615,835	51
								114,090	19

Table 6 (continued)

								156,150	24
			195						
66,000	33	496,400		12,000	6	43,556	17	48,819	10
242,990	102								
179,520	27								
								493,995	170
75,133	27							1,255,169	57
84,000	14								
				50,000	15				
				12,000	2			642,227	55
38,500	14								
35,625	48								
								252,904	21
						181,100		5,000,490	247
							46	20,192	49
								2,764,145	69

Table 7

DVM Student Tuition and Fees - First Year (Class of 2013)

School	Tuition		Fees		Room & Board	
	Res	NR	Res	NR	Res	NR
AUB	13,402	39,226			8,972	8,972
UCD		12,245	24,507	24,507	12,870	12,870
CSU	17,362	45,462	1,496	1,496	8,346	8,346
COR	26,500	39,500			8,100	8,100
FLA	20,667	20,667	2,458	23,525	8,170	8,170
UGA	12,770	12,770	1,460	1,460	8,046	8,046
ILL	19,240	37,704	2,754	2,754	11,526	11,526
ISU	15,682	37,260	895	895	8,550	8,550
KSU	16,614	39,101	1,484	1,484	6,752	6,752
LSU	12,640	12,640	2,059	26,259	14,347	14,347
MSU	21,174	44,658	504	504	10,224	10,224
MIN	22,146	42,190	2,608	2,608	9,612	9,612
MIS	14,147	35,232	1,511	1,511	9,998	9,998
UMO	16,662	16,662	1,118	16,834	9,550	9,550
NCSU	9,352	32,115	1,558	1,558	11,248	11,248
OSU	25,095	58,533			8,172	8,172
OKL	12,390	29,670	2,110	2,110	7,650	7,650
ORE	16,989	34,314	1,638	1,638	8,352	8,352
PENN	30,902	39,486	2,912	2,912	15,500	15,500
PUR		23,268	17,018	17,018	8,710	8,710
TENN	17,444	39,612	922	1,222	10,060	10,060
TAMU	10,188	20,988	4,186	4,186	9,986	9,986
TUF	36,468	39,426	400	400	12,000	12,000
TUS	18,850	27,600	360	360	9,261	9,261
VMR	15,299	37,101	3,116	3,506	8,600	8,600
WSU	18,332	45,342	838	838	9,492	9,492
WES	40,105	40,105	40	40	11,766	11,766
WIS	16,697	24,769	1,018	1,018	8,740	8,740
US AVG	19,120	33,130	3,159	5,626	9,807	9,807
CLG	10,410		230			
ONT	6,182	51,196	1,217	1,217		
MON	4,338					
PEI	9,348	49,528	696	696	7,200	7,200
SKW	6,750		925		6,000	

NR = Non-resident; refers to all out-of-state/at-large applicants

Table 7 (continued)

Books & Equipment		Personal		Transportation		Health	
Res	NR	Res	NR	Res	NR	Res	NR
3,329	3,329	2,446	2,446	2,286	2,286		
3,856	3,856	2,362	2,362	1,788	1,788	1,959	1,959
1,404	1,404	1,804	2,504			1,950	1,950
900	900	5,910	5,910			1,590	1,590
1,600	1,600	650	650	540	540	2,484	2,480
1,250	1,250	2,300	2,300	270	270		
1,800	1,800					584	584
1,044	1,044	4,235	4,235	1,322	1,322		
2,800	2,800	1,425	1,425	2,630	2,630	1,920	1,920
3,600	3,600	2,918	2,918	1,830	1,830	1,267	1,267
1,588	1,588	2,500	2,500	1,566	1,566	1,390	1,390
1,588	1,588	2,000	2,000	750	750	2,408	2,408
8,500	8,500			4,676	4,676		
1,570	1,570	6,400	6,400				
2,259	2,259	3,111	3,111	1,100	1,100		
3,780	3,780	1,260	1,260	2,088	2,088	1,620	1,620
1,360	1,360	2,440	2,440	1,810	1,810		
1,603	1,603	2,469	2,469				
1,500	1,500	3,360	3,360			2,642	2,642
1,160	1,160	1,760	1,760	2,630	2,960		
2,996	2,996	3,676	3,676	2,050	2,050	1,500	1,500
2,142	2,142	2,187	2,187	664	900		
775	775	3,300	3,300			3,276	3,276
1,654	1,654	4,107	4,107	1,985	1,985	500	500
1,100	1,100	1,760	1,760	1,600	1,600	2,300	2,300
1,200	1,200	2,108	2,108	1,434	1,434	1,262	1,262
2,629	2,629	4,953	4,953	3,572	3,572	1,164	1,164
1,320	1,320	2,500	2,500	580	580	1,770	1,770
2,154	2,154	2,844	2,871	1,770	1,797	1,755	1,755
3,000							
1,000	1,000						1,512
1,100							
2,000	2,000	1,800	1,800	1,000	2,000	320	829
3,000				1,800			

Table 7 (continued)

	Other		TOTAL STUDENT EXPENSES	
Res	NR		Res	NR
			30,435	56,259
			47,342	59,587
			32,362	61,162
			43,000	56,000
1,040	1,040		37,609	58,672
	24,200		26,096	50,296
2,760	2,760		38,664	57,128
2,500	2,500		34,228	55,806
1,000	1,000		34,625	57,112
			38,661	62,861
600	600		39,546	63,030
1,230	1,230		42,342	62,386
			38,832	59,917
			35,300	51,016
			28,628	51,391
2,844	2,844		44,859	78,297
100	100		27,860	45,140
			31,051	48,376
			56,816	65,400
			31,278	54,876
			38,648	61,116
			29,353	40,389
			56,219	59,177
12,176	12,176		48,893	57,643
3,500	3,500		37,275	59,467
1,000	1,000		35,666	62,676
525	525		64,754	64,754
150	150		32,775	40,847
2,263	3,830		42,872	60,970
657			14,297	0
			8,399	54,925
			5,438	0
2,000	2,000		24,364	66,053
120			18,595	0

Table 8

Students Not Holding a DMV Degree and Not Enrolled in DVM Program

School	Associate Degree				BS			
	Total	Min.	%Min.	FN	Total	Min.	%Min.	FN
AUB			0.0%				0.0%	
UCD			0.0%		8	1	12.5%	
CSU			0.0%		144	24	16.7%	
COR			0.0%				0.0%	
FLA			0.0%				0.0%	
UGA			0.0%				0.0%	
ILL			0.0%				0.0%	
ISU			0.0%				0.0%	
KSU			0.0%				0.0%	
LSU			0.0%				0.0%	
MSU	15	1	6.7%		65	2	3.1%	
MIN			0.0%				0.0%	
MIS			0.0%				0.0%	
UMO			0.0%				0.0%	
NCSU			0.0%				0.0%	
OSU			0.0%				0.0%	
OKL			0.0%				0.0%	
ORE			0.0%				0.0%	
PENN			0.0%				0.0%	
PUR	32	2	6.3%		17		0.0%	
TENN			0.0%				0.0%	
TAMU			0.0%		1746	556	31.8%	68
TUF			0.0%				0.0%	
TUS			0.0%				0.0%	
VMR			0.0%				0.0%	
WSU			0.0%				0.0%	
WES			0.0%				0.0%	
WIS			0.0%				0.0%	
CLG			0.0%				0.0%	
ONT			0.0%				0.0%	
MON			0.0%				0.0%	
PEI			0.0%				0.0%	
SKW			0.0%				0.0%	

Min = Minority students   FN = Foreign National students

Table 8 (continued)

MS or Equivalent				MPVM			
Total	Min.	%Min.	FN	Total	Min.	%Min.	FN
19	2	10.5%	17			0.0%	
5	1	20.0%				0.0%	
79	11	13.9%				0.0%	
1		0.0%				0.0%	
29	2	6.9%	1			0.0%	
		0.0%				0.0%	
		0.0%				0.0%	
5		0.0%				0.0%	
14	2	14.3%	7			0.0%	
2		0.0%	2			0.0%	
13	1	7.7%	3			0.0%	
1		0.0%				0.0%	
6	1	16.7%	1			0.0%	
2		0.0%	1			0.0%	
		0.0%				0.0%	
		0.0%				0.0%	
5		0.0%				0.0%	
		0.0%				0.0%	
		0.0%				0.0%	
3		0.0%	1			0.0%	
		0.0%				0.0%	
13	1	7.7%				0.0%	
14	2	14.3%				0.0%	
3	1	33.3%	2			0.0%	
6		0.0%	3			0.0%	
		0.0%				0.0%	
		0.0%				0.0%	
5		0.0%	3			0.0%	
3		0.0%				0.0%	
31		0.0%				0.0%	
5		0.0%				0.0%	
2		0.0%				0.0%	
3		0.0%				0.0%	

Table 8 (continued)

	MPH				PhD		
Total	Min.	%Min.	FN	Total	Min.	%Min.	FN
		0.0%				0.0%	
19	7	36.8%		21	7	33.3%	4
		0.0%		23	2	8.7%	
		0.0%		18	1	5.6%	6
		0.0%		2		0.0%	1
		0.0%				0.0%	
		0.0%				0.0%	
		0.0%		3		0.0%	
3		0.0%		20	1	5.0%	14
		0.0%		4		0.0%	2
		0.0%		1		0.0%	1
3	1	33.3%				0.0%	
		0.0%		2		0.0%	
19	5	26.3%	2	4		0.0%	
		0.0%				0.0%	
6		0.0%		3	1	33.3%	2
		0.0%		7	4	57.1%	1
		0.0%				0.0%	
		0.0%				0.0%	
		0.0%				0.0%	
		0.0%		1		0.0%	1
		0.0%		16	6	37.5%	
		0.0%				0.0%	
		0.0%				0.0%	
		0.0%		5		0.0%	3
		0.0%				0.0%	
		0.0%				0.0%	
		0.0%		8		0.0%	4
		0.0%		2		0.0%	
		0.0%		5		0.0%	
		0.0%		2		0.0%	
		0.0%		1		0.0%	
		0.0%		5		0.0%	

Table 9

DVM Student Attrition (Classes 2009-2012)

School	CAUCASIAN					MINORITY					GRAND TOTAL
	YR1	YR2	YR3	YR4	TOTAL	YR1	YR2	YR3	YR4	TOTAL	
AUB	1				1					0	1
UCD		1	2	1	4					0	4
CSU	1	2	1	1	5			1		1	6
COR			1		1					0	1
FLA	1				1					0	1
UGA	3	2			5					0	5
ILL	1				1					0	1
ISU		4			4					0	4
KSU		2			2					0	2
LSU			5		5					0	5
MSU	2		1		3					0	3
MIN	1		1		2					0	2
MIS	1				1					0	1
UMO	10	3	1		14					0	14
NCSU	1				1	2				2	3
OSU	2	2	2	1	7		1			1	8
OKL	3				3	1				1	4
ORE	1		1		2					0	2
PENN	2				2					0	2
PUR	2	2	1		5					0	5
TENN	1		1		2					0	2

Table 9 (*continued*)

TAMU	4	2			6					0	6
TUF		1			1	2				2	3
TUS	1				1	1	2	1		4	5
VMR		1	1		2	1	1			2	4
WSU		1			1					0	1
WES	1	3			4	2	2			4	8
WIS				1	1	1				1	2
US Total	38	27	18	4	87	10	6	2	0	18	105
CLG					0					0	0
ONT					0					0	0
MON		1	1		2					0	2
PEI					0					0	0
SKW					0					0	0
Can. Total	0	1	1	0	2	0	0	0	0	0	2
Grand Total	38	28	19	4	89	10	6	2	0	18	107

*Canadian institutions do not all report ethnic identity.

For the purpose of this table, students may be reported under the Caucasian column.

Table 10
Reasons for DVM Student Attrition (Classes 2009 - 2012)

School	CAUCASIAN			MINORITY			GRAND TOTAL
	Low Grades	Other	Total	Low Grades	Other	Total	
AUB	1		1			0	1
UCD			0			0	0
CSU	1	4	5		1	1	6
COR		1	1			0	1
FLA	1		1			0	1
UGA	2	3	5			0	5
ILL		1	1			0	1
ISU	1	3	4			0	4
KSU			0			0	0
LSU	1	4	5			0	5
MSU	3		3			0	3
MIN		2	2			0	2
MIS		1	1			0	1
UMO			0			0	0
NCSU	1		1	2		2	3
OSU	5	2	7	1		1	8
OKL	3		3	1		1	4
ORE	1	1	2			0	2
PENN		2	2			0	2
PUR	4	1	5			0	5

Table 10 (*continued*)

TENN		2	2			0	2
TAMU	5	1	6			0	6
TUF	1		1	2		2	3
TUS	1		1	4		4	5
VMR	2		2	2		2	4
WSU	1		1			0	1
WES	2	2	4	1	3	4	8
WIS	1		1	1		1	2
US Total	36	31	67	14	4	18	85
CLG			0			0	0
ONT			0			0	0
MON	1	1	2			0	2
PEI			0			0	0
SKW			0			0	0
Can. Total	1	1	2	0	0	0	2
Grand Total	37	32	69	14	4	18	87

*Canadian institutions do not all report ethnic identity.
For the purposes of this table, students may be reported under the Caucasian column.

Table 11

DVM Student Raw Test Scores - First Year (Class of 2013)

School	Mean GRE Verbal	Mean GRE Quantitative	Mean GRE Analytical	Other Test	Mean
AUB	485	619			1104
UCD	575	712	5	GRE	431
CSU	522	643	5	GRE-General	540
COR	609	732			
FLA	524	679			
UGA	528	588	5	GRE BIO	1109
ILL	500	655	4		
ISU	490	630	4		
KSU	522	667	5	GRE	
LSU	500	641			
MSU	517	656			
MIN	520	650			
MIS	454	577	4	GRE	1031
UMO				GRE (general)	1098
NCSU	525	653	4		1182
OSU					1206
OKL	477	628	4	Biology Subject Test	560
ORE	65	62	54		60
PENN	578	710			
PUR	471	632	5	Purdue	
TENN	495	646	4	GRE Verbal + Quan	1141
TAMU	490	654	4		
TUF	610	710	5		
TUS	407	509	4		
VMR	560	690	5	GRE	
WSU					57
WES	479	642	5		
WIS	541	692	5		
CLG					
ONT					
MON					
PEI					
SKW					

Table 12

Profile of Professional First Year DVM Students (Class of 2013)

School	Mean Pre-Vet GPA	Grade Scale	Mean Age	Years of Pre-Professional Prep (Number of Students with ...)						Number of Students with Degrees			
				Mean Yrs. of Prep.	2yr	3yr	4yr	5yr	6(+)yr	No Degree Complete	BS/BA	MS/MA	PhD
AUB	3.53	A=4.0	23.00	6.00		14	38	20	23	16	76	2	1
UCD	3.53	A=4.0	24.00	4.50	3	27	55	21	27	9	124	14	2
CSU	3.60	A=4.0	25.00	5.05	2	2	39	40	55		115	20	3
COR	3.67	A=4.0	23.00	3.90	7	35	23	18	9		88	1	3
FLA	3.51	A=4.0	24.60	4.40			58	20	10		79	9	
UGA	3.54	A=4.0	23.00	4.00		10	52	21	19	7	88	7	
ILL	3.54	A=4.0	24.20	4.00		6	109		3	6	109	3	
ISU	3.53	A=4.0	23.80	4.10	2	5	121	17	4	4	137	8	
KSU	3.60	A=4.0	23.80	4.30		17	46	27	22	30	78	4	
LSU	3.77	A=4.0	23.70	4.31	3	18	31	14	18	28	59		
MSU	3.66	A=4.0	23.00	2.00		13	89	4		13	89	3	1
MIN	3.54	A=4.0	24.00	4.00		10	34	20	28	10	76	6	
MIS	3.48	A=4.0	24.56	4.75		12	24	27	17	22	48	10	
UMO	3.74	A=4.0	23.00	4.00						20	88	2	

227

Table 12 (continued)

NCSU	3.70	A=4.0	23.46	4.20					7		72	5	2
OSU	3.52	A=4.0	21.50				72			1	128	8	1
OKL	3.56	A=4.0	24.00	4.50		12	42	11	17	25	54	3	
ORE	3.62	A=4.0	23.30	5.20		5	21	11	17	2	52	10	2
PENN	3.61	A=4.0	23.79	4.23			100	10	12		110	2	
PUR	3.56	A=4.0	22.50	4.00		13	47	9		14	54	2	
TENN	3.60	A=4.0	23.70	3.94		10	57	11	7	6	77	2	
TAMU	3.67	A=4.0	21.24	4.45	5	32	51	18	22	4	114	13	2
TUF	3.66	A=4.0	25.00			2	75	2	8		77	9	
TUS	3.22	A=4.0	24.00		3	28	35				35	6	
VMR	3.65	A=4.0	22.00		1		68	15	11	1	88	5	
WSU	3.58	A=4.0	24.70	4.50		1	92	5		1	97	13	
WES	3.26	A=4.0	26.00							2	82	6	3
WIS	3.61	A=4.0	23.00	4.53		10	36	21	13	8	66	7	
US Avg	3.57		23.60	4.30		13	57	16	17	11	84	3	
CLG	3.36	A=4.0	24.27	4.17		7	11	4	6	15	12	13	2
ONT			23.20		22	36	35	5	1	18	68	2	
MON			21.17	2.96	49	9	12	10	4	47	14	1	
PEI			25.00	5.00	8	3	27	14	11	14	48	2	
SKW				4.49	1	21	30	11	14	34	40	2	1

Table 13

Total DVM Student Enrollment by Ethnic Identity (Class of 2013)

School	African Amer.		Hispanic		Asian		Pacific Islander		Native American		Alaskan Native		Multi-Ethnic		Other Minority	
	m	f	m	f	m	f	m	f	m	f	m	f	m	f	m	f
AUB		3		1		1				1						
UCD		2	1	5	3	18		1	1					4	1	1
CSU	1	2	4	7		5				2						
COR	1	1	2	4		4								2		
FLA	1	1	2	10	1	1										
UGA	2	2	1	2		1				1						
ILL		3	1	3		2									1	2
ISU				2												1
KSU			1	5	4	5	1			3				3		
LSU	1	1	1	3		1										
MSU	1	1		1		4				1						
MIN		1	1			1				1						
MIS	1			2		1			1							
UMO			1	2		2										
NCSU	2	6		4		1				1						
OSU			1	5	1	3		1		2						2

229

Table 13 (continued)

OKL							2	3									
ORE	1		3												3		
PENN	1	2	5	2	2	2											4
PUR	1	2	2	3	2	2		1									
TENN			2	2				1									
TAMU	3	8	11	2	2	2					1				1		2
TUF	1	4	2	1	1	1					1						
TUS	3	25	1	1	1	1											
VMR	1	4			1	4										2	
WSU	1	4	1	1	4			2			1						
WES	2	1	2	6	2	11					1				2		
WIS	1	1	5	5									1	2			
US Total	15	55	32	90	23	83	1	5	0	4	19	0	0	1	14	4	12
CLG																	
ONT																	
MON																	
PEI																	
SKW																	
Can	0	0	0	0	0	0	0	0	0	0	0	0	0	0	0	0	0
Total	15	55	32	90	23	·83	1	5	0	4	19	0	0	1	14	4	12

*N/A - Not available; Canadian institutions do not all report ethnic identity.

Table 13 (continued)

Minority Total			N/A*		Caucasian		Foreign National		Grand Total		
m	f	all	m	f	m	f	m	f	m	f	all
0	6	6			28	61			28	67	95
6	31	37		7	18	74			24	112	136
5	16	21	1	9	19	88			25	113	138
3	11	14	3		14	61			20	72	92
4	12	16			12	60			16	72	88
3	6	9			23	70			26	76	102
2	10	12			20	88			22	98	120
0	3	3	5	5	34	74	1	1	40	83	123
6	13	19			23	69		1	29	83	112
2	8	10	1	4	19	52			22	64	86
1	7	8		5	12	80	1		14	92	106
1	3	4			20	73			21	76	97
2	3	5			20	55			22	58	80
1	4	5	1	3	21	87			23	94	117
2	12	14	1	5	12	47			15	64	79
2	13	15			36	91			38	104	142

Table 13 (continued)

2	6	8			18	56			20	62	82
1	5	6	1		10	37			12	44	56
4	12	16	2		24	78		1	30	92	122
3	7	10			10	49			13	57	70
1	4	5			13	67			14	71	85
8	19	27	1		20	84			29	103	132
3	6	9			13	64		1	16	71	87
5	26	31		5	8	17	2	3	15	51	66
2	5	7			24	67			26	72	98
2	7	9	2	4	21	62			25	73	98
7	16	23	4	28	15	31		1	26	76	102
2	7	9	2	2	15	55			17	64	81
80	278	358	22	80	522	1797	4	9	628	2164	2792
0	0	0	9	22					9	22	31
0	0	0	23	83			3	3	26	86	112
0	0	0		15	15	69			15	69	84
0	0	0	9	33			3	18	12	51	63
0	0	0							0	0	0
0	0	0	41	138	15	69	6	21	62	228	290
80	278	358	63	218	537	1866	10	30	690	2392	3082